D0450158

Praise for *The Great American Heart Hoax*

"Michael Ozner, MD, a visionary and compassionate cardiologist, has been on a single-minded mission for the past three decades. His goal? To prevent, reverse, and ideally eliminate the raging epidemic of heart disease that continues to claim so many lives.

Unlike most cardiologists today, Dr. Ozner lives by his well-known philosophy of 'prevention not intervention.' In *The Great American Heart Hoax*, Dr. Ozner distills more than thirty years of clinical practice, giving you an easy-to-follow 10-step program to avoid the degenerative risks of heart disease. In addition, Dr. Ozner provides practical information and tools on working with your doctor to obtain optimal health, thereby avoiding unnecessary surgery, tests, and countless bottles of medication. As you read, Dr. Ozner is your personal guide through the most practical method for achieving cardiac health, providing you with the inside information you need to become a more responsible, more informed partner in your own care.

I strongly urge you to stop whatever you are doing and immediately start reading the life-saving information contained in this book. What you learn will change the way you live your life."

—PHILIP SMITH,
Editor-in-Chief, *Life Extension Magazine*

Praise for Dr. Ozner's Previous Book, *The Miami Mediterranean Diet*

"I strongly recommend Dr. Ozner's book, *The Miami Mediterranean Diet*, for anyone who is interested in living a long and healthy life. This book is a concise, no-nonsense approach for heart disease prevention. With so many fad diets that are here today and gone tomorrow, finally there is a clinically proven and sensible approach, as Dr. Ozner provides practical dietary and lifestyle guidelines for defeating heart disease."

—BARRY T. KATZEN, MD,
Medical Director, Baptist Cardiac & Vascular Institute of Miami

"The current medical literature is replete with articles confirming what Dr. Ozner has been advocating for many years—that prevention is the best treatment for heart disease. In his book, *The Miami Mediterranean Diet*, he outlines a strategy that, combined with an exercise program, has allowed me to reduce my weight, my blood pressure, and my cholesterol. I have a greater sense of well-being and I feel that I will live a longer and healthier life."

—JERROLD YOUNG, MD

"In *The Miami Mediterranean Diet*, Dr. Michael Ozner not only makes a compelling argument for the importance of the Mediterranean diet and lifestyle for overall health, but gives a comprehensive guide for ways to incorporate this diet into all of our lives. Research has clearly shown that those who follow a life-long Mediterranean diet and lifestyle are giving themselves the best insurance for a healthy life and now Dr. Ozner brings that to our shores."

—RANDOLPH P. MARTIN, MD,
Director of Noninvasive Cardiology, Emory University Hospital

"A valuable resource from preventive cardiologist Michael Ozner providing heart healthy dietary information, sample meal plans, and an exciting array of recipes."

—NANETTE K. WEGNER, MD,
Professor of Medicine (Cardiology), Emory University School of Medicine

"This book is a direct path to the visceral pleasure of well-prepared food and cardiovascular health. *The Miami Mediterranean Diet* provides a sane alternative to the faddist and extremist diets that lead to short-term weight loss and long-term weight gain."

—JOSEPH IZZO, JR., MD,
Professor of Medicine & Pharmacology,
State University of New York at Buffalo
Clinical Director of Medicine, Erie County Medical Center, Buffalo,
New York

"I wholeheartedly endorse the Mediterranean diet, a way of eating that has been in existence for thousands of years. *The Miami Mediterranean Diet* is based on this way of life, encouraging a balanced, well-nourished food plan including whole grains, fresh fruits and vegetables, and lower fat intake. Following Ozner's stated food plan, coupled with caloric control and daily exercise, can lead to both weight loss and a healthy heart. The recipes are easy to produce and generate delicious meals; no one would feel deprived adhering to the stated plan."

—KAREN LIEBERMAN, PhD, RD,
Professor and Chair, The Hospitality College
Johnson & Wales University, Florida Campus

The Great American HEART HOAX

LIFESAVING ADVICE YOUR DOCTOR SHOULD TELL YOU ABOUT HEART DISEASE PREVENTION

(BUT PROBABLY NEVER WILL)

Michael Ozner, MD

BENBELLA BOOKS, INC.

Dallas, Texas

BenBella Books, Inc.
6440 N. Central Expressway, Suite 503
Dallas, TX 75206
www.benbellabooks.com
Send feedback to feedback@benbellabooks.com

Printed in the United States of America
10 9 8 7 6 5 4 3 2

Library of Congress Cataloging-in-Publication Data is available for this title.

Proofreading by Stacia Seaman
Cover design by Melody Cadungog
Text design and composition by John Reinhardt Book Design
Printed by Bang Printing

Distributed by Independent Publishers Group
To order call (800) 888-4741
www.ipgbook.com

For special sales contact Robyn White at robyn@benbellabooks.com

To contact Dr. Michael Ozner: www.drozner.com

To my wife Christine
and my children
Jennifer and Jonathan:
You are my heart and soul.

Acknowledgments

I WOULD LIKE TO THANK my many patients and colleagues who have given me the inspiration and motivation to write *The Great American Heart Hoax*.

I am especially grateful to Charles Hennekens, MD, for taking the time to review *The Great American Heart Hoax*. Dr. Hennekens, the first Eugene Braunwald Professor of Medicine at Harvard Medical School and the first Chief of Preventive Medicine at Brigham and Women's Hospital in Boston, has contributed immensely to the field of cardiology and epidemiology for decades, and I am honored to have him write the foreword to this book.

I would also like to thank Philip Smith, editor-in-chief at *Life Extension Magazine*, for his continuous help and guidance. In addition I would like to thank Dale Kiefer and Cathy Lewis for their important contributions.

I am fortunate to work with the medical education department at Baptist Hospital of Miami. They have helped me organize and implement an annual cardiovascular disease prevention symposium highlighting recent advances in heart disease prevention. This meeting has become one of the premier symposiums in America dedicated to the prevention and treatment of cardiovascular disease.

I am also grateful to Glenn Yeffeth, publisher of BenBella Books, for his unwavering support. Special thanks to all those at BenBella who have been a pleasure to work with: Leah Wilson (senior editor), Laura Watkins, Adrienne Lang, Yara Abuata, and Robyn White.

Finally, and most importantly, I would like to thank my wife, Christine Ozner, RN, who has provided me with endless love, guidance, and encouragement.

Contents

Foreword

NOBODY WOULD DISAGREE THAT, at present, the life expectancy of men and women living in the United States is the greatest it's ever been. This is a result chiefly of declines in mortality from coronary heart disease and stroke, the leading contributors to deaths from cardiovascular disease. During the last decade, major contributions have been made in the fight against cardiovascular disease by early diagnosis and medical treatment of patients by their health care providers. Yet it is also true that many patients seem to prefer the prescription of pills or costly interventions to the proscription of harmful lifestyles.

Surgical intervention of cardiovascular disease using coronary artery bypass grafting or angioplasty with stent placement in the unstable patient appear to have net clinical benefits, optimally as adjuncts to medical therapies. Nevertheless, intervention with a scalpel or a stent is potentially avoidable for the vast majority of patients with stable coronary disease.

Eugene Braunwald, MD, Professor Emeritus at Harvard Medical School, was perhaps the doyen of cardiovascular medicine of the second half of the twentieth century. He was also my boss, and I felt honored to serve as the first Eugene Braunwald Professor of Medicine at Harvard Medical School. In a 1977 editorial in the *New England Journal of Medicine*, Professor Braunwald wrote with clairvoyance, "An even more insidious problem is that an industry is being built around heart bypass surgery.... [T]his rapidly growing enterprise is developing a momentum of its own, and as time passes it will be progressively more difficult to curtail it...."

Based on the foregoing, *The Great American Heart Hoax* makes a unique contribution to patients as well as their health care providers. Dr. Ozner's "lifesaving advice" is always prudent, rational, and plausible, and with it, readers are forewarned and forearmed to take a proactive approach to the prevention and treatment of cardiovascular disease, which is and will remain far and away the leading cause of death in the United States and is now the leading cause of death in the world.

There is proof beyond a reasonable doubt that coronary heart disease is not an inevitable consequence of an increasing lifespan and, indeed, is preventable. In this regard, Dr. Ozner's book should be welcome to anyone facing the complex medical and public health challenges of the twenty-first century.

CHARLES H. HENNEKENS, MD, DRPH
Voluntary Professor, University of Miami
Miller School of Medicine
Clinical Professor, Nova Southeastern University
Sir Richard Doll Research Professor, Florida Atlantic University,
Boca Raton, Florida

Introduction

Primum Non Nocere
(Above all, do no harm!)

—Hippocrates

WITHIN THE PAGES OF THIS BOOK you will learn the dirty little secret that is undermining the credibility of the most sophisticated health care system the world has ever known. You'll discover how this broken paradigm for medical care leads to unnecessary heart surgery and is threatening to bankrupt our economic system.

According to recent statistics, heart disease is the leading cause of death in the United States. An indiscriminate killer, heart disease has occupied this top spot for decades. And it's joined by stroke, another vascular disease, in the number three spot. America is not alone in this; heart disease is consistently a leading killer throughout much of the industrialized world, according to statistics reported by the World Health Organization. But take heart. I'm here to share the good news: *Heart disease is preventable.* We know how to halt its progression, and even reverse it—all without expensive, invasive procedures or costly brand name prescription medications.

America spends at least $60 billion a year on invasive cardiovascular care. Even in these days of escalating national debt and unbalanced budgets, that's a staggering amount of money. And shockingly, evidence suggests that much of it is being squandered on high-risk, expensive procedures that have not been proven to either save lives or prevent heart attacks. Studies show that these now-common cardiac procedures— including coronary artery angioplasties, stent placements, and coronary bypass surgeries—are of dubious value, adding little in terms of long-term health outcomes, and sometimes even making things worse than if they hadn't been performed at all. America has 5 percent of the world's population, yet we perform half of the world's bypass surgeries and stent placements. And countries that spend a fraction of what we do on heart surgery have fewer per capita heart attacks and fewer heart-related deaths! Cardiovascular care is an almost obscenely lucrative industry in America, and evidence abounds that financial concerns may be distracting hospitals and physicians from focusing on what should be their primary concern: what's truly best for the patient.

The American Heart Association reports that 80 million men and women suffered from cardiovascular disease in 2005. Many of those unfortunate individuals experienced severely reduced quality of life, enduring symptoms that include intermittent to constant chest pain, the inability to walk, breathlessness, and countless drug side effects, among other troubling symptoms. As heart disease worsens, doctors are often forced to prescribe an increasing number of drugs to alleviate escalating symptoms—medications that present the risk of dangerous drug interactions. And despite the billions spent on cardiovascular medicine annually, nearly a million men and women in America over the age of eighteen die each year of heart disease.

Clearly, we have a problem. But it doesn't have to be this way. We don't *have* to resign ourselves to lives of increasingly clogged arteries and ever-mounting risk of heart attack or stroke. Nor must we resign ourselves to dependence on expensive medications, or submit to surgeries that don't work. There *is* an alternative to invasive procedures, costly surgery, and an ever-declining quality of life.

The solution to heart disease costs little, and provides benefits in abundance. And it doesn't involve wishful thinking, unattainable goals, or trendy—but untested—methods. It's a solution that works. In my work as an experienced, well-trained, board-certified cardiologist and a Fellow of both the American Heart Association and the American College of Cardiology, I've seen countless numbers of patients not only avoid worsening heart disease, but actually improve their health and quality of life; I know what I'm talking about. And I've shared my passion for the subject of heart disease prevention with my fellow physicians and other health care professionals in countless lectures across America and around the world.

But you needn't just take my word for it, either. There's decades' worth of solid, published scientific evidence to prove that the methods outlined in this book actually work. And these methods can be implemented readily by virtually anyone—anyone, that is, who wants to live longer, feel better, and get more out of life.

In Part I, we'll look at how heart disease develops, how we treat it, and the evidence that our current treatment methods don't work. Then in Part II, I'll tell you what does work—and why. You'll learn the ten steps that can empower you to take charge of your health and confidently say "no thanks" to invasive, expensive, and ultimately futile medical procedures.

Heart disease doesn't have to be our nation's leading killer—and by reading this book, you're taking the first step toward helping to change that.

PART ONE

THE PROBLEM

CHAPTER 1

The Heart Surgery Hoax

The philosophies of one age have become the absurdities of the next, and the foolishness of yesterday has become the wisdom of tomorrow.

—Sir William Osler, 1902

I
T WAS A FEW HOURS BEFORE DAWN in late 1979. I was fresh out of my cardiology fellowship, in my first year of practice, and instead of sleeping, I was working frantically on an emergency room patient who had woken suddenly in the middle of the night with chest pain and then collapsed. By the time he arrived in the ER, he had no pulse or blood pressure and his pupils were fixed and dilated. The EKG monitor showed a flat line.

Medications, multiple shocks from the defibrillator, and even the bedside insertion of a pacemaker failed to revive him, and after an hour of CPR, one of the nurses informed the patient's wife and two young daughters that it was unlikely he would make it. But finally, after using a long needle to inject epinephrine directly into his heart, a blip appeared on the heart monitor and his pulse and blood pressure returned!

Once the patient was stable I went out and gave his wife the good news. She'd been preparing herself to hear her husband was dead, and instead I told her he was going to live. She cried, tears of joy and relief, and hugged me. And after an extensive hospital stay, her husband left the hospital alert and happy to be alive—and understandably concerned with making sure what had just happened would never happen again.

The patient, Jim, a thirty-nine-year-old businessman with a strong family history of premature coronary heart disease and mildly elevated cholesterol and blood pressure, sat down with me shortly after. The first thing I did was give him a copy of the forty-page heart disease prevention manual I'd just recently finished putting together: "The Optimal Diet & Lifestyle for Cardiovascular Health."

A few weeks earlier, I'd come home from a long day at work and read an article that completely changed the way I looked at the practice of cardiovascular medicine. Between 5 A.M. that morning, when I'd arrived at the hospital for work, and just before midnight, when I'd finally left for the day, I'd treated half a dozen heart attack patients in the ER and performed an angioplasty late in the evening. All I wanted was to eat something, catch up a little on my professional reading, and collapse into bed. What I picked up to read that night was an article about the Seven Countries Study, a landmark twenty-year study by Dr. Ancel Keys at the University of Minnesota.

The data from the study revealed that countries in the Mediterranean basin had a radically lower incidence of many diseases we took for granted in the Western world, including diabetes, cancer, and notably, heart disease. The average middle-aged Greek man had a *90 percent lower risk* of dying from a heart attack than the average middle-aged American. What Dr. Keys had concluded was that the explanation for this discrepancy could be found in the dietary habits and lifestyle of the region. And the traditional Mediterranean diet and lifestyle was particularly associated with a low risk of coronary heart disease. "If some developed countries can do without heart attacks," Dr. Keys asked, "why can't we?"

I was stunned. The people living in the Mediterranean basin were getting better results with a knife and fork than we were with all our fancy equipment and advanced technologies! The next day I dove into research, and when I finally came up for air, I was convinced that we were going about heart disease treatment the wrong way. The solution wasn't surgery; it wasn't bypasses and balloon angioplasties and stents. We couldn't just treat the effects of heart disease. We had to treat the cause: the diet and lifestyle factors that led to heart disease in the first place. We needed *prevention*, not intervention.

I was so convinced, in fact, that what I had learned could not only prevent but also halt and even *reverse* heart disease, that I immediately sat down in front of my typewriter and typed out nearly forty pages of information on prevention I believed my patients desperately needed to know. Those were the same pages I gave to Jim, just recovered from his cardiac near-death experience and serious about preventing a subsequent attack. And I began handing these pages to all of the other patients who came in to see me.

In a matter of months I was starting to hear from people across the country, who'd talked to the cousin of a friend of a patient of mine, and wanted a copy of "that Mediterranean diet program" for themselves. And more importantly, I began to notice that my patients who followed my advice just weren't having heart attacks anymore. Back then, it wasn't uncommon to have two, three, even four of your patients in the ER with a heart attack on a given day. And suddenly, mine weren't having any—including those patients who'd had procedures in the past and had been judged likely to return to the operating room. Clearly, something was happening. And the longer this went on, the more sure I became that my prevention plan was working—and the more I believed the treatment the medical community was providing for its patients was not only less effective than prevention, it was actually detrimental to the patients who received it.

The Numbers Tell the Story

More than 1.5 million angioplasties and coronary bypass surgeries are done annually in the U.S., which makes heart surgery among the most commonly performed surgical procedures for both men and women. Although heart surgery can be lifesaving, the truth is that surgery benefits only a small fraction of the millions of patients who undergo these operations. For the majority—an estimated 70 to 90 percent—these procedures are at best unnecessary. In fact, except for a minority of patients, bypass surgery and angioplasty have *never* been shown to prolong life *or* prevent heart attacks. And while American patients are seven times more likely to undergo coronary angioplasty and bypass surgery than patients in Canada and Sweden, the number of Canadians and Swedes who die from cardiovascular disease is *nearly identical* (per capita) to the number of people who die from heart disease in this country.

It sounds unbelievable, but it's true. We're spending billions of dollars every year on risky procedures that have never been shown to benefit the majority of patients, or make a significant difference in the overall mortality rate.

It concerns me that countless patients are subjected every day to unnecessary surgeries. But what makes it worse is that these procedures can be harmful. Although doctors often hasten to assure their patients that these procedures are time-tested and safe, all invasive surgery carries risk.

In fact, the mortality rate for bypass surgery ranges from 3 to 5 percent. This may sound insignificant initially, but when you consider that half a million people undergo these procedures every year, 3 to 5 percent quickly adds up: to 15,000 to 25,000 lives lost a year. Additionally, an estimated 25 to 30 percent of angioplasties fail, requiring patients to repeat the procedure. And eventually many of these angioplasty patients will also require bypass surgery.

The mortality rate isn't the only worrying statistic associated with bypass surgery. Up to 80 percent of patients may experience cognitive difficulties after surgery, something that can be especially devastating to elderly patients, who may already be experiencing problems with memory and other early signs of cognitive decline. People who undergo bypass surgery are nearly four times more likely to suffer a subsequent stroke at the time of surgery than if they had elected not to go under the knife. They are also vulnerable to post-surgical infections. Nor are coronary angioplasty and stent placement risk-free; complications include heart attack, stroke, aneurysm at the puncture site, infection, and the potential need for emergency bypass surgery.

Other possible adverse effects of heart bypass surgery include:

- Heart attack or stroke at the time of surgery
- Accelerated atherosclerosis (up to tenfold) in the artery that has been bypassed
- Post-operative depression
- Severe anxiety
- Infection, including wound infection, lower extremity infection at the site where the vessel for the bypass is harvested, and sepsis (dangerous infection in the bloodstream)
- Delayed healing of the wound
- Inflammation of the pericardium (the thin tissue lining the heart)
- Blood loss, requiring transfusion

- Kidney failure
- Repeat bypass surgery due to closed bypass grafts—note that repeat surgery is even more problematic, with reported mortality rates of 15 to 20 percent!

The other adverse effect of heart bypass surgery is on your wallet; in some cases it has led to financial ruin. The cost of heart bypass surgery can range from $40,000 to more than $100,000. And the surgery itself can lead to prolonged disability and loss of income, making it even more difficult to pay medical bills.

Contrast this with the cost of following a heart-healthy lifestyle: none!

An Important Disclaimer

I'm not saying that all heart surgery is a hoax. Far from it! Over the past thirty years, tremendous strides have been made in the surgical treatment of many once-fatal heart problems.

Indeed, heart surgery is a lifesaver for many, many patients. Today, heart surgeons perform heroic work, saving babies with once-fatal congenital heart defects. Cardiothoracic surgeons can repair an aorta that dissects or ruptures, or replace diseased heart valves, or save a patient in the throes of a massive heart attack who, in earlier eras, would surely have died. Heart transplants are all but routine now, and they've saved many people whose hearts have failed them for any number of reasons. Interventional cardiologists are able to open occluded coronary arteries in patients in the midst of a heart attack, restoring blood flow and saving heart muscle. And these are just a few examples of the wonderful advancements we've made in cardiac surgery, advances that represent unparalleled achievements in our ability to save lives.

Atherosclerosis-related conditions that do warrant surgical intervention include disabling chest pain, despite maximal medical therapy and lifestyle changes; severe blockage of the left main coronary artery; critical blockages of all the major coronary arteries in patients with a weak heart muscle; and unstable coronary syndromes, such as an evolving heart attack.

Don't mistake my intent: my concern isn't with cardiac intervention that's appropriate. My concern's with the sheer number of inappropriate and unnecessary procedures that are performed—procedures that subject stable patients with coronary artery disease to needless risk when they would be far better served in other ways.

So What's the Hoax?

The hoax is that even though the medical community knows these things, most of us haven't changed the way we practice cardiac medicine. Most heart disease patients are sold a bill of goods by a cardiology industry that has a vested interest in making sure that as many people as possible are treated with expensive surgical procedures, rather than with far less costly lifestyle changes, and/or medications. We tell patients we'll "fix" them with surgery, but we don't—and sometimes we only make things worse.

By now, you should be asking a couple of questions. First, why *doesn't* heart surgery work? Second, and more important, if heart surgery doesn't work, why do we keep doing it?

To answer these questions, we need to begin by understanding the details of what heart disease is, and how it develops.

CHAPTER 2

Heart Disease—
It's Not Worth Dying For!

The heart is a tough organ: a marvelous mechanism that, mostly without repairs, will give valiant service up to a hundred years.

—DR. WILLIS POTTS, heart surgeon (1959)

WHAT WE CALL cardiovascular disease encompasses a wide range of conditions that affect the heart and vascular system, from high blood pressure (hypertension), to coronary artery disease, to heart failure, heart attack (myocardial infarction), peripheral arterial disease, aneurysm, and stroke, among others. All are manifestations of disease within the heart or within the literally thousands of miles of blood vessels in our bodies. Throughout the industrialized world, cardiovascular disease is the number one killer of men and women. And it's accelerating in some developing countries, too. The specter of cancer frightens people, but consider this: In the U.S. alone, heart disease is responsible for about 40 percent of all deaths, taking more lives each year than all forms of cancer combined.

Common risk factors for heart disease include advancing age, sedentary lifestyle, *high* levels of low-density lipoprotein cholesterol (LDL cholesterol) and triglycerides, *low* levels of high-density lipoprotein cholesterol (HDL cholesterol), smoking, obesity (particularly "central," or abdominal, obesity), high levels of fibrinogen, elevated C-reactive protein (a marker of inflammation), a family history of heart disease, high blood pressure, and chronic mental stress. And because men are likely to be stricken by heart disease earlier in life, being male is also a risk factor. (Women don't get off the hook, however. They're about ten times as likely to die of cardiovascular disease as breast cancer, and 60 percent of all deaths from stroke occur in women.) Obviously, some of these factors cannot be avoided—gender, and family history, for example. But others, such as smoking or chronic inactivity, clearly can.

The majority of heart disease is related to something called atherosclerosis, the "hardening" of the arteries through chronic inflammation due to fatty deposits in the artery wall. Healthy arteries are tough while still remaining flexible and elastic. Atherosclerosis gradually destroys this crucial elasticity. When arteries harden and narrow, they can block the flow of vital oxygen and nutrient-rich blood to the heart, brain, and other organs. Unfortunately, for a majority of men and about half of all women with atherosclerosis, the first indication that they have this condition is heart attack or sudden cardiac death. Atherosclerosis may take decades to develop, and its progression is stealthy. It is this insidious development of atherosclerosis, and how to prevent it, that is the primary focus of this book.

The best way to understand heart disease and atherosclerosis is to take a look at the way a healthy heart and circulatory system function. So let's back up for a moment, review the fundamental anatomy and physiology of this remarkably complex yet elegant organ and delve more deeply into what transforms a healthy cardiovascular system into a dysfunctional one.

The Healthy Heart

During an average lifetime, the heart will beat faithfully, about 2.5 billion times, at a rate of about seventy-two beats per minute. The heart begins beating long before we are born, but when it stops, in the absence of immediate medical intervention, so do we. Despite the enormous workload placed on the heart, it is an amazingly robust organ, capable of squeezing oxygen-rich blood to the farthest reaches of the body while simultaneously receiving oxygen-depleted blood and then shunting it to the lungs for oxygenation before beginning the cycle all over again. And so it goes, moment by moment, day in and day out, seldom noticed and requiring little or no thought on our part.

It is tempting to think that hard work—running fast for a mile, for example, or lifting something heavy—would put a strain on the heart. After all, hard exercise can easily raise the pulse, or heartbeats per minute, well above 120. But nature designed us for daily exercise, and working harder actually improves the functionality of the heart and the many blood vessels that carry vital nutrients, oxygen, and waste products throughout the body. Together, the heart, blood, arteries (mostly carrying oxygen-rich blood), veins (mostly carrying oxygen-depleted blood), smaller arterioles, tiny capillaries, and even smaller venules form the cardiovascular system, also known as the circulatory system.

Heart muscle (or cardiac muscle) is a type of involuntary muscle found nowhere else in the body. Specialized nerve cells provide a coordinated series of electrical impulses that travel across the various chambers, orchestrating steady, rhythmic contractions, perfectly timed to meet the body's needs and maximize the heart's blood-pumping efficiency.

The right atrium, located at the top of the heart, receives oxygen-depleted blood from the body, delivered via the body's largest vein, the vena cava. It's squeezed into the right ventricle (the larger, more muscular lower chamber on the right side of the

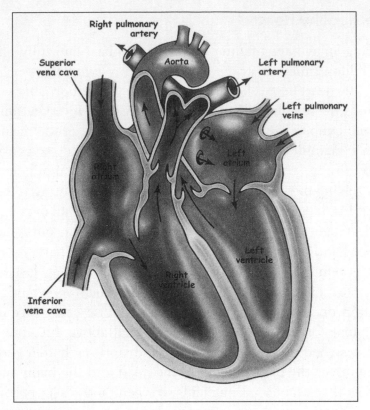

Figure 1: Cross-section of the heart.

heart) and is subsequently ejected, through the pulmonary artery, to the lungs.

This pulmonary circulation allows waste carbon dioxide gas, generated as the body uses oxygen to turn calories into energy, to be exchanged for oxygen in the lungs. Freshly oxygenated blood is then shunted back to the heart, via the pulmonary vein, where it enters the left atrium, moves to the left ventricle, and is squeezed forcefully into the aorta, the body's largest artery. The aorta quickly branches into other arteries, which in turn supply blood to the rest of body. Because it must do the lion's share of the work, the left ventricle is noticeably larger and more muscular than the right.

Various heart valves comprise the final structures of importance in the heart. Located between chambers and between the left ventricle and the aorta, the valves prevent leakage and backwash of blood during pumping, thus increasing the heart's efficiency.

Understanding Heart Disease

The key to understanding cardiovascular disease is understanding the structure and physiology of the blood vessels—arteries, veins, arterioles, capillaries, and venules—themselves. Many things can go wrong with the heart, but barring defects present at birth, relatively uncommon attacks by bacteria and other microbes, or trauma, the heart is remarkably robust. Like any muscle, however, it requires a great deal of freshly oxygenated, nutrient-rich blood to work. To that end, a network of coronary arteries entwines the organ, delivering a constant supply of blood to the heart's muscular walls so that the heart can continue its tireless beating.

And therein lies the source of the vast majority of problems encountered in cardiovascular medicine. When these supply routes become blocked, the cardiac muscle becomes starved for oxygen and nutrients, and quickly dies. This blockage is referred to as coronary artery disease, and is the end result of the long-term, ongoing disease known as atherosclerosis. The result of this blockage—cutting off blood supply to the heart muscle, often is accompanied by acute pain and a heart attack.

Atherosclerosis precipitates heart attack by generating "plaques"—swelled accumulations of white blood cells and cholesterol inside the artery wall—that rupture and cause sudden blockage due to clot formation. When the plaque lining a coronary artery develops a fissure or tear and ruptures, blood platelets quickly adhere to the rupture site, forming a blood clot. The clot either blocks blood flow completely or breaks loose and travels to a smaller branch of the coronary artery, where it may lodge and create a blockage. When coronary arteries become blocked, portions of the heart muscle begin to starve, and may eventually die.

Although not all heart attacks are fatal, none are trivial. Heart muscle does not grow back; dead heart tissue impairs heart function indefinitely. And when a clot forms elsewhere, such as in the proximal aorta, it may travel to the brain, precipitating a stroke.

Our Arteries Are Not Pipes

My first year in medical school, I remember sitting in vascular biology class listening to a lecture on why heart attacks occur. The prevailing wisdom at the time was that the progressive buildup of cholesterol deposits in the artery wall eventually culminated in an atherosclerotic plaque—a collection of cholesterol-laden cells that became walled off and covered by a thick fibrous cap. It was felt that this plaque grew in size until it eventually choked off the inside of the artery, shutting off blood flow. Heart attack was the result. If this process occurred in the brain it caused a stroke.

This explanation seemed logical—a progressive accumulation of sludge led to a stoppage of blood flow in our pipes and bingo!, a heart attack resulted. After all, isn't this what happens to a sink drainpipe when it backs up? So the solution seemed obvious: Since heart attacks were nothing more than a plumbing problem with the "pipes" in the body, you just needed to get rid of the sludge. If your pipes at home get clogged, you call the plumber. He arrives, "snake" in hand, and clears the obstruction by performing "surgery" on your pipes. Why couldn't a doctor do the same for your arteries? And if your doctor couldn't successfully "snake out" the clog, a surgeon could always just bypass it, adding a new pipe through which blood could flow freely. Sounds simple. Makes sense. Why not?

I'll tell you why not. Our arteries are not pipes! The plumbing analogy never made sense to me. As a medical student studying vascular biology I was amazed at the complexity of our blood vessels. The vascular tree is an active, living organ that expands and contracts in response to different stimuli, not a network of rigid metal conduits. Its walls are permeable—and cholesterol doesn't just build up inside an open space like so much drain-pipe sludge.

During my student days there was a tremendous interest in lowering fat and cholesterol, the presumed cause of the sludge backing up our arterial pipes. Cholesterol-lowering was the new cardiac buzzword, and new medications were being developed to accomplish the task, first resins, then niacin, and ultimately the superstar of them all, statins. The American Heart Association convened a conference in 1960 and declared war on fat. Since blockages were caused by cholesterol (a specific kind of fat), surely lowering the fat and cholesterol in our diet would decrease the buildup of sludge and lower the incidence of heart attack. But despite this "war," millions of Americans continued to die. The frequency of death from heart attack even went up! How could this be? How could the heart attack rate continue to increase despite the national campaign to lower fat and cholesterol?

This was our first inkling that we may have gotten it wrong. Evidence suggested that there had to be more to atherosclerosis than just cholesterol and fat. In 1948, an ambitious U.S. government-sponsored study of the long-term causes of cardiovascular disease had been launched in Framingham, Massachusetts. Over the decades, investigators had accumulated huge amounts of data regarding the lifestyle and dietary habits of a large group of individuals who had, at the beginning of the study, been free of disease. When the data from the Framingham study revealed that the cholesterol level in most heart attack victims was no different than that of those who didn't have a heart attack, the mystery deepened. The data did reveal, however, that people with very high cholesterol readings experienced a higher incidence of heart attack and those with very low readings were largely spared from heart attack. Clearly cholesterol was involved somehow. The question was how.

Understanding the Role of Cholesterol in Heart Disease

Cholesterol is not inherently evil. In fact, the body manufactures its own supply—it's a necessary, fundamental building block of cell membranes and other compounds needed by the body, such as steroid hormones. For this reason, it is undesirable to eliminate *all* cholesterol from the bloodstream. But cholesterol is also obtained from the diet. In the absence of a genetic defect which causes an individual's body to over-produce cholesterol, the primary source of excess cholesterol, especially "bad" LDL cholesterol, can be traced to the diet, and to lack of exercise, which suppresses the "good" HDL cholesterol that helps remove excess LDL cholesterol.

If you've had a cholesterol panel done, you know that what doctors normally test for are total cholesterol, LDL cholesterol, HDL cholesterol, and triglycerides. You know that LDL is "bad" cholesterol and HDL is "good" cholesterol, and that a high level of triglycerides is a risk factor for heart disease. But what does all of that really mean?

LDL and HDL aren't actually types of cholesterol at all—they're particles responsible for carrying cholesterol through the body. Cholesterol can't travel through the bloodstream on its own; it needs LDL, HDL, and other lipoproteins to transport it where it needs to go. You can think of cholesterol-carrying particles (lipoproteins) as moving through the bloodstream like cars traveling down the highway; they carry cholesterol the same way cars do people. When your doctor measures your LDL and HDL cholesterol, he's actually measuring the volume of cholesterol found inside the LDL and HDL particles in your blood—the number of passengers inside the cars, not the number of cars on the highway.

The reason we call LDL cholesterol "bad" cholesterol is because LDL particles are the particles that enter our artery walls, where the cholesterol becomes trapped and leads to atherosclerosis. Here, too, thinking of cholesterol-carrying particles as cars is useful. When the highway is busy, cars are more likely to take alternate routes to avoid the traffic; similarly, the more cholesterol particles in the bloodstream, the more likely cholesterol particles are to leave the bloodstream and enter the artery walls.

HDL particles, in contrast, seek out cholesterol inside the artery walls and act like straws, sucking out the cholesterol and transporting it to the liver for disposal—which is why we call HDL cholesterol "good" cholesterol. HDL cholesterol also has important antioxidant and anti-inflammatory functions.

Triglycerides affect heart disease risk in a more indirect way. Triglycerides are a kind of fat that serves as a back-up energy source for the body. When we digest food, fats are broken down by our gastrointestinal tract and repackaged as triglycerides before being taken to fat cells for storage. But the gastrointestinal tract is not the only place fats are repackaged as triglycerides. Fatty acids that end up in the liver are also repackaged as triglycerides, and transported to cells via a lipoprotein called VLDL because, like cholesterol, triglycerides can't travel on their own.

When one of these triglyceride-rich VLDL particles encounters a cholesterol-rich LDL particle, a swap takes place. When they go their separate ways, the VLDL particle is the cholesterol-rich particle, and the LDL particle is the triglyceride-rich particle. The real trouble begins when that triglyceride-rich LDL particle comes across a particular kind of enzyme, which burns away the triglycerides inside. As a result, the LDL particle shrinks. LDL and HDL particles vary in size, depending on several factors. Some of the factors are genetic; others are environmental, a result of lifestyle choices. While all LDL particles are able to enter the artery wall, small particles are *more likely* to do so than large particles. Returning to our metaphor: smaller LDL particles are like compact cars that can squeeze into parking spots SUVs (larger LDL particles) can't. This is what makes high levels of triglycerides so dangerous: their effect on LDL particles. The same swap-and-shrink occurs in HDL particles, but the end result there is that the smaller HDL particle becomes less capable of removing cholesterol from the artery wall.

We know all this now. Back then we were only just discovering how much we didn't know about cholesterol—including how much cholesterol was too much. Dr. William Castelli, a noted preventive cardiologist and former director of the Framingham Study, frequently mentioned the "150 club" in talking about the study's results. He noted that none of the study subjects with a total cholesterol of less than 150 had suffered a heart attack. It turned out that the typical American's cholesterol was so far above healthy levels that what we assumed was normal was actually too high; when I started my cardiology practice in 1979, a *normal* cholesterol level meant up to 300 mg/dl! Other studies supported what the Framingham Study had found: Populations around the world with practically nonexistent coronary heart disease and heart attack had total cholesterol readings in the 120s.

This discrepancy between our previous beliefs about safe cholesterol levels and reality was disturbing: If we were wrong about that, what else were we wrong about? Even though medications had been effective in lowering cholesterol and reducing the risk of heart attack, there were still large numbers of patients in clinical trials who were suffering heart attacks. Evidently, cholesterol wasn't the only problem.

Atherosclerosis: The Root of the Problem

Not all heart problems are related to atherosclerosis. But in the vast majority of cases, atherosclerosis is the ultimate culprit.

Atherosclerosis, recall, is the hardening of the artery due to a buildup of atheromatous plaques inside the artery wall. Atheromatous plaques typically have three components: the atheroma, a flaky, yellowish clump of white blood cells; a layer of oxidized cholesterol crystals; and in older plaques, areas of calcification at the outer base. You can think of these plaques as the arterial equivalent of a pimple on your skin: just like a pimple, they become inflamed, grow, and ultimately rupture, releasing pus-like contents.

The development of an atheromatous plaque begins when cholesterol enters the artery wall, but there are two chief biological responses that are essential to plaque formation: oxidation, and inflammation.

Oxidation

Oxidation is a chemical reaction involving one of the most basic things our bodies need to live: oxygen. We all know that we need oxygen to survive, but we don't always know why exactly that is. Oxygen is a necessary part of turning the food we eat into the energy we need to live, through a process called cellular respiration. Cellular respiration is a pretty efficient process, but it does produce a potentially dangerous byproduct: oxygen free radicals.

"Free radical" is a term used for any molecule with an uneven number of electrons. Electrons, you may remember from high school chemistry, are nearly always arranged in pairs. Molecules with unpaired electrons are unstable, always seeking out the extra electron they need to become complete—which they accomplish by stealing an electron from another molecule. That theft by free radicals is referred to as oxidation.

This is the same process that occurs in a cut apple when its inside turns brown, or in a pipe when it rusts. We just can't see it with our eyes when it happens inside our bodies, causing tissue damage at the cellular level that affects even cell DNA.

Atherosclerosis begins when cholesterol particles squeeze through the barrier of endotheliel cells and into the lining of the artery walls (or intima), but the real trouble starts when that cholesterol comes into contact with free radicals inside the artery wall. The free radicals steal electrons from the cholesterol particles, oxidizing them.

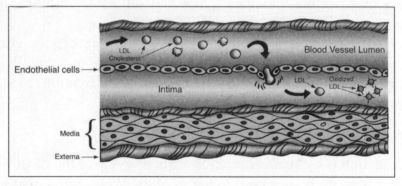

Figure 2: LDL cholesterol particle squeezes through to the lining of the artery wall and becomes oxidized.

This triggers an immune response; our body attacks the oxidized cholesterol as if it were a foreign invader. It is this immune response, inflammation, that then leads to the development, progression, and rupture of plaques.

Inflammation

The inflammatory response is designed to protect us from the virus, bacteria, and other foreign invaders that find their way into our bodies. It consists of four basic parts: first, it attacks the threat; second, it engulfs (and tries to dissolve) the threat; third, it isolates the threat from the rest of the body; and fourth, it extrudes whatever is left of the threat and the leftover inflammatory cells.

What happens when you get a splinter in your finger provides an excellent example. The immune system recognizes the splinter—and the bacteria it inevitably carries with it—as a hostile foreign invader. White blood cells are rapidly dispatched to the scene. Once there, they engulf and dissolve the splinter, while temporarily protecting the body from the potentially lethal threat by walling it off from its surroundings. Finally, after the threat is taken care of, they break down the wall, extruding anything left of the original splinter, and allow the area to heal.

When a cholesterol particle enters the artery wall and becomes oxidized, it becomes a "splinter" in the wall of the artery. Inflammatory cells sense the danger and come rushing to the scene.

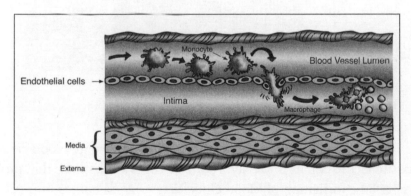

Figure 3: Oxidized cholesterol is engulfed by white blood cells.

The oxidized LDL cholesterol is quickly engulfed by specialized white blood cells called monocytes, and is walled off by smooth muscle cells, which produce a thick fibrous cap of collagen over the working white blood cells. The white blood cells, in the meantime, secrete several noxious substances. The most important for our discussion here are proteinases and tissue factor—the two enzymes responsible for plaque rupture and the subsequent blood clot.

Plaque Rupture and Blood Clot

Proteinases are enzymes that break down the collagen that forms the plaque's thick fibrous cap. The proteinases eat away at the collagen like tiny pac-men until the cap is weak enough for the plaque to rupture, spilling its contents into the vessel, where it comes in contact with the blood.

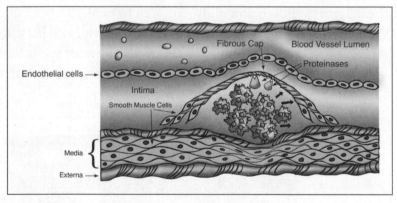

Figure 4: Proteinases eat away at the plaque's thick fibrous cap.

This is where the other substance secreted by white blood cells, tissue factor, comes into play. Tissue factor is a substance that promotes the formation of blood clots. When blood comes into contact with tissue factor, it clots instantly. Platelets then come rushing to the scene to contribute to the clot, which can result in partial or complete blockage of the blood vessel at the clot site.

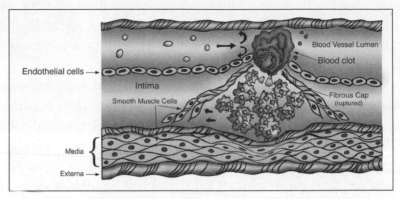

Figure 5: Tissue factor from the ruptured plaque and platelets cause blood to clot, blocking blood flow in the artery.

Not every plaque ruptures. Some plaques are perfectly stable. But while those may eventually grow large enough to restrict blood flow and cause chest pain, the real threat is unstable plaques—the ones that rupture and cause a clot.

There are three possible outcomes of a sudden rupture of an atherosclerotic plaque and the subsequent blood clot:

1. The blood clot is small and produces no symptoms.
2. The blood clot is moderate to large in size and partially blocks blood flow to the heart muscle, causing the patient to experience chest pain.
3. The blood clot blocks blood flow completely, resulting in a heart attack and the death of heart muscle cells.

Our bodies can dissolve blood clots; it's an ability that's essential to our survival. But the body must maintain a delicate balance between forming clots and dissolving them. A body that dissolves clots too aggressively can bleed to death; a body that dissolves clots too sluggishly risks blocking its own blood flow unnecessarily. Given this natural ability, it's possible that you have had several plaques rupture in your coronary arteries just today, but because your body was able to dissolve the clots, you remained blissfully unaware. It's only when such clots are not disposed of—when they result in heart attack or stroke—that we notice them.

When it comes to the likelihood of plaque rupture, small plaques are actually *more* likely to rupture, and thus become a danger, than larger ones—an important and often overlooked point, because patients are often sold on the idea of stents or bypasses based on information about large, scary blockages. There are a couple of reasons for this. First, small blockages are more common than large blockages. Second, small blockages often lack the thick calcified cap that protects and covers the plaque in large blockages, so they rupture more easily. Finally, large blockages foster the development of something called collateral blood vessels—new vessels that spontaneously develop, forging a path around the blockage—whereas small blockages, since they don't significantly restrict blood flow, do not.

Like water in a stream that's been partially dammed, blood naturally tries to find a way around any blockage in a vessel. Blood often finds that way around through tiny blood vessels that form, circumvent the plaque, and then reconnect with the original path, the coronary artery. As a blockage grows, cutting off blood flow gradually, more and more blood is forced onto that alternate path, until that path is fully developed. As a result, the heart muscle is able to receive the oxygenated blood it needs, despite the blockage in the original vessel.

Conventional wisdom dictates that if a coronary artery is completely blocked, the heart muscle must have been damaged. However, it is not uncommon to discover an occluded artery in patients with no history of chest pain or heart attack. The reason is these collateral blood vessels do on their own what surgeons do when they perform a surgical bypass—which is why I like to call this phenomenon "natural" heart bypass. Our best explanation for this phenomenon is that we all possess these collateral vessels, but they lie dormant until they receive a chemical signal indicating that they need to activate. Then they spring to life.

Dutch researchers commented on this process in a recent article on the subject in *The International Journal of Cardiology*, noting, "Collaterals exert a protective effect on outcome in a broad spectrum of patients." Swiss researchers published a report in 2007 on a ten-year follow-up study of 845 men and women with coronary artery disease. Patients with low "collateral flow index"—patients who had few, or poorly functioning, collaterals—were statistically more likely to die of cardiac disease than patients with good collateral flow. In fact, patients with good collateral circulation were 75 percent less likely to die of heart attack than patients with poor collateral circulation.

The collateral vessels only develop, however, in response to blockages that have grown slowly, over time. They don't appear instantaneously; blood clots from ruptured plaques block blood flow too quickly for this natural bypass process to take place. So while your body offers some protection from large ruptured plaques by forming these collateral vessels, they're useless if a small blockage suddenly ruptures and causes a heart attack. Collaterals simply don't occur in small, non-obstructive plaques.

So What Do We Do About It?

We've looked at how the cardiovascular system is supposed to work; we've looked at our blood vessels, and how they respond to cholesterol; we've looked at how atheromatous plaques develop, and their potential consequences.

What we need to look at now is the measures cardiac medicine currently recommends for treating heart disease. What can we do about unstable plaques, whether large or small? How do we keep them from rupturing, or even forming in the first place?

CHAPTER 3

Understanding Heart Surgery

THE FIRST SCIENTIFIC STUDY OF THE HEART was done in the second century A.D., by Greek physician Galen of Pergamum, who determined through animal dissection and inference (as he was hampered by restrictions against human dissection) that arteries and veins had different functions, and between them carried blood throughout the human body. His observations, both right and wrong, prevailed until the Renaissance, when Leonardo da Vinci gave us the very first accurate, detailed drawing of the human heart. And in 1628, William Harvey's *An Anatomical Study of the Motion of the Heart and of the Blood in Animals* revolutionized the way scientists thought about the heart and circulatory system yet again, for the first time correctly describing in detail the way the circulatory system works.

Other advancements soon followed. In the early eighteenth century, English clergyman and scientist Stephen Hales became the first to measure blood pressure. By 1816 French physician Rene T. H. Laennec had invented the stethoscope, better enabling doctors to listen to the sounds made by the beating heart and thus improving diagnosis of heart ailments. At the dawn of the twentieth century Dutch physiologist Willem Einthoven developed the electrocardiogram, or EKG, which is used to this day to look at the heart's electrical activity.

By the mid-twentieth century, cardiac medicine was progressing rapidly. In 1951 American surgeon Charles Hufnagel developed a plastic valve to repair a defective aortic valve, and in 1961 the first external cardiac massage was successfully used to restart a human being's heart. In 1964 the first heart transplant was performed at the University of Mississippi Medical Center. The dying patient received a chimpanzee heart, which beat for about ninety minutes before failing. In 1965 American surgeons Michael DeBakey and Adrian Kantrowitz implanted the first mechanical devices to assist a diseased heart, and in 1967 Christiaan Barnard, a South African surgeon, performed the first transplant of a human donor heart. The recipient, Louis Washkansky, survived for eighteen days before succumbing to pneumonia. In 1982 American surgeon William DeVries implanted the world's first permanent artificial heart into a patient. The device had been engineered by American physician Robert Jarvik, who improved upon an earlier design developed by Paul Winchell in 1963. The Jarvik-7, as it was known, enabled patient Barney Clark to live for an additional 112 days.

For the most part, the quest for a suitable artificial replacement for a living heart has met with disappointing results, but as more and more people suffer and die from heart disease, medical science perseveres, looking for new and better ways to save lives.

Aside from replacing damaged hearts, however, what other options does cardiac medicine offer us? What has it learned about the best ways to keep heart disease patients from needing a replacement heart in the first place? How do we treat heart disease today? When a patient goes to see a cardiac doctor, they are usually classified as needing one of two kinds of preventative care: primary preventative care or secondary preventative care. The patient who comes in with no clear evidence of atheromatous plaques, but who has a family history of heart disease and may have high cholesterol, high blood pressure, or other risk factors, is given primary preventative care. The focus is on reducing risk factors.

The patient who comes in with established plaques—perhaps he or she has had an ultrasound or CAT scan that showed blockages, or perhaps he or she has had a previous heart attack —is given secondary preventative care. This includes working to reduce risk factors, but especially in the last few decades, it also usually means something else: surgery.

Surgical Intervention

Surgery's role in cardiac medicine often begins even before any blockage is established. When a doctor suspects possible narrowing of one or more of the coronary arteries due to atherosclerosis, he may order a catheterization, the insertion of a long thin tube into a chamber or vessel of the heart, as an investigational tool. The catheter is usually put in through the femoral artery, located in the groin, and snaked through the blood vessels until it reaches the heart. There, it injects iodinated contrast dye into the coronary arteries to determine if a blockage is present.

If a coronary artery blockage is confirmed, the doctor may either address it then, or else note the location for a separate, future procedure. If the doctor does address it then, he does so with a procedure called balloon angioplasty—a vascular intervention to widen a narrowed or occluded artery.

In balloon angioplasty, a balloon-tipped catheter is inserted into the vessel, threaded to the site of the blockage, and then inflated, crushing (or rather, displacing) the plaque against the wall of the artery and opening the vessel for optimal blood flow. The balloon is then deflated and removed.

In most cases today, a flexible, expandable wire-mesh tube— a stent—will also be inserted. The stent is wrapped around the angioplasty balloon before it is threaded to the site of the blockage. When the balloon inflates, the stent expands to line the interior of the vessel. When the balloon deflates, the stent remains in place, holding the vessel open. This is done to improve the chances that the vessel will remain this way. Newer drug-coated stents are often used to further discourage blockage from re-developing.

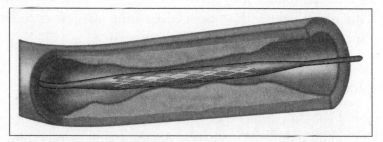

Figure 6: The balloon-tipped catheter is inserted, with the stent wrapped around the outside.

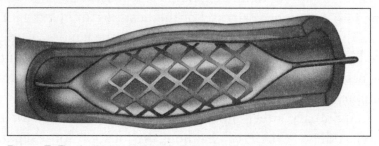

Figure 7: The balloon is inflated, displacing the plaque against the artery wall as it expands.

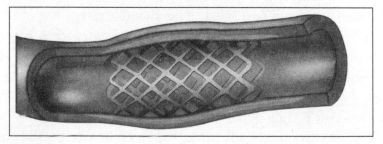

Figure 8: The catheter is removed, leaving the stent in place to hold the unblocked artery open.

Another option for dealing with a serious blockage is to go around it: to take a piece of vessel from another part of the body and graft it surgically to the blocked artery in such a way that the blood is then able to bypass the blockage entirely.

In the early 1960s an Argentine doctor by the name of Rene G. Favaloro immigrated to the U.S., where he began groundbreaking work on revascularization, or repairing blood flow in blocked blood vessels, at the Cleveland Clinic. In 1967 he and his team pioneered the first coronary bypass operation, drawing on established research on the bypass of blockage in the legs. They removed a vein from a patient's leg and used it to create a new route around the obstructed portion of the patient's right coronary artery. This ground-breaking operation soon became known as coronary artery bypass graft surgery (CABG), or more commonly, coronary bypass surgery.

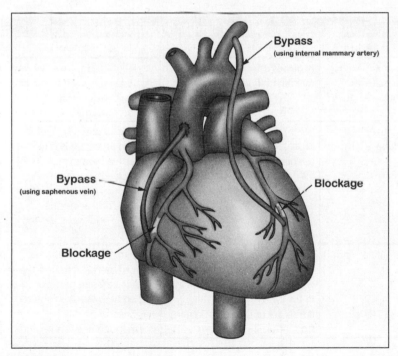

Figure 9: Types of coronary artery bypass.

In coronary bypass surgery, the chest is opened, and vessels are harvested for use in the bypass. In some cases, the heart is stopped. One end of the graft vessel is sewn into the artery on the outside of the blockage; the other is sewn onto the aorta. If necessary, the heart is restarted. Then the chest is closed and the patient taken to the intensive care unit. Bypass surgery is clearly the most serious and invasive of these options, involving major surgery and requiring approximately four days of recovery time in-hospital alone. In contrast, catheterization, angioplasty, and stent placement are considered minimally invasive procedures, since access to the interior of the body is obtained through a distant blood vessel. This doesn't mean they are risk-free, however. They aren't even outpatient procedures; most patients stay at least overnight afterward for observation.

Atherosclerosis-Related Cardiac Surgery/Procedures		
Procedure	What It Does	How It Works
Coronary Artery Bypass Graft (CABG) Surgery	Bypasses artery blockage to maintain blood flow.	Vessel grafted from elsewhere in the body is used to bypass a blocked portion of a coronary artery or arteries.
Coronary Angioplasty	Mechanically widens an obstructed coronary artery by opening and/or widening the inside of the vessel.	A catheter with an inflatable balloon at the tip is threaded through a blood vessel in the groin or arm until it reaches the heart. The balloon is inflated, displacing the blockage and widening the artery.
Stent Placement	Holds open arteries that have been newly unblocked and widened through angioplasty. In the case of coated stents, it also discourages blockage from returning.	An expandable wire-mesh tube is inserted through the cardiac catheter and placed at the point where angioplasty has been performed. The tube is expanded and left behind.

Since heart surgery's tentative beginnings just half a century ago, we've come to rely on it as the gold standard for heart disease treatment. It's become big business in America, supporting multiple other industries and bringing in millions of dollars in profit every year.

But while the advances that have accompanied heart surgery's growth certainly seem impressive, we've overlooked something very important, something we'll look at in-depth in the next chapter: whether or not, for the vast majority of patients, any of it actually *works*.

CHAPTER 4

Why Bypass Surgery and Angioplasty Seldom Work and Why We Keep Doing Them Anyway

Surgery is always second best.
If you can do something else, it's better.

—Heart surgeon DR. JOHN KIRKLIN, Mayo Clinic, 1963

I WAS A YOUNG CARDIOLOGIST IN TRAINING when Andreas Gruentzig developed balloon angioplasty, and I'll never forget the excitement that rippled through the cardiology community when Dr. Gruentzig first displayed the X-ray images showing before-and-after pictures of blocked and unblocked coronary arteries. The results in the "after" photos looked incredible, and like many of my colleagues, I was amazed. Finally, we felt, we had a new, effective weapon in the fight against heart disease.

After finishing my cardiology fellowship, I went to Baptist Hospital in Miami and assisted with the first balloon angioplasty there, with the same amazing results. But it wasn't long before I started having doubts. I saw more and more patients, who had supposedly undergone successful procedures, coming back—again and again—for repeat angioplasties. And the same thing was happening in hospitals all over the country. It soon became obvious to me that angioplasty was not the panacea we had all hoped for. But I was one of the few who saw it.

In those early days many felt that it would be cardiologists with their catheters, not surgeons with their scalpels, who would "fix" the problem of clogged arteries. Initially no one even bothered to conduct clinical trials on whether coronary balloon angioplasty actually prevented heart attacks or saved lives. "Why do clinical trials? It's obvious that opening a blocked coronary artery is beneficial and will help the patient," one physician remarked at an annual meeting of cardiologists.

A feeding frenzy had begun. Once bypass surgery was developed, an entire industry devoted to supporting it followed. Surgical programs mushroomed, fellowship programs proliferated, cardiac anesthesiologists were trained, operating rooms were built, and hospitals and cardiac centers were constructed. Angioplasty, too, spawned its own industry. Interventional cardiology became its own specialty; cardiology programs mass-produced cardiologists specially trained to perform the lucrative procedure.

Along the way, hospitals discovered that the fastest way to financial security—prosperity, even—was to expand their menu of cardiac services and ancillary services: surgical suites, and radiology departments offering scans and tests. Soon every hospital in America was building "cardiac cath labs" to cash in. Hospitals without cath labs were finding it difficult to stay in business; it was either join the party or shut down. But as one interventional cardiologist once told me, "What could be better? In a matter of minutes I can open up a blocked artery and fix the patient, and make millions of dollars a year."

Cardiac care centers are cash cows, bringing in huge profits that help finance less lucrative areas of medicine. It's been estimated that we spend at least $60 billion per year on interventional cardiac medicine. If all that interventional medicine worked, the cost would be worthwhile. The trouble is, it doesn't.

The Evidence

There may not have been many clinical studies done at first on the effectiveness of new heart disease treatments, but researchers have been busy since, putting coronary bypass surgery, angioplasty, and stents up against non-surgical heart disease treatment in rigorous studies. In every case, the surgical solutions came up short.

Coronary Bypass Surgery

Three major studies performed in the late 1970s and early 1980s clearly proved that for the majority of patients, bypass surgery is no more effective than conservative medical treatment. These three studies were the Veterans Administration Cooperative Study (the VA Study), the Coronary Artery Surgery Study (CASS), and the European Coronary Artery Surgery Study (EuroCASS). These studies began in 1977 with the VA study, which compared patients who underwent bypass surgery with similar patients who received only medical therapy. Unexpectedly, the results showed that, with the exception of a small subset of patients, bypass surgery did *not* lower the death rate *or* prevent heart attacks.

And how did the cardiology juggernaut react? Rather than step back and take a second look at these practices and procedures, they just criticized the study. Physicians opined that the findings were somehow wrong; that, in fact, the opposite must surely be true. So our nation's official health agency, the

National Institutes of Health, launched the CASS. Like the VA Study, the CASS found that a majority of patients who underwent bypass surgery did not live significantly longer or have fewer heart attacks than those who did not undergo surgery. And the European CASS reached similar conclusions.

All three of these were well-designed studies, published in major peer-reviewed medical journals. And while these studies were done in the 1970s, the results are not outdated. The cardiac medications available then were much less effective than the ones we use today. Statins, for example, did not exist in the '60s and '70s. So if anything, similar studies conducted today would be expected to find non-surgical treatment even *more* effective and still *more* preferable to surgery. In addition, the patients from the original studies have been tracked and subjected to follow-up studies over the past two decades. These follow-up studies show the same results: *bypass surgery does not prolong life or prevent heart attacks in the majority of patients.*

One thing bypass surgery *has* been shown to do is reduce chest pain. But recent studies indicate that the reason for this may have less to do with the bypass of the blockage, and more to do with the act of cutting into the patient's chest—which often destroys pain receptors around the heart, logically leading to less pain. If this is the case, it could be that bypass surgery affects the *ability* to feel pain as much as what was causing the pain in the first place. As well, bypass surgery is not the only, or even best, way to reduce chest pain. (We'll talk more about effective alternate treatments in later chapters.)

Angioplasty

The studies on angioplasty delivered even worse news: angioplasty didn't show any benefit either. If anything, unless the patient was in the midst of a heart attack, the opening of a blocked coronary artery with a balloon catheter resulted in a *worse* outcome compared to management through medication.

One of the trials most hotly contested by angioplasty proponents was published in 1999. This was the Atorvastatin Versus Revascularization Treatment (AVERT) Trial, the first study designed to pit aggressive, cholesterol-lowering statin drug therapy against balloon angioplasty in patients with coronary artery blockages. These patients had chest pain but were neither unstable nor in the throes of a heart attack. The results, which were published in the *New England Journal of Medicine* in 1999 by Dr. Bertram Pitt and colleagues, found to everyone's surprise that the lives of patients treated with angioplasty *were not* significantly prolonged compared to similar patients who received medical therapy alone, nor did they suffer fewer heart attacks. In fact, aggressive cholesterol-lowering through medication was associated with a decrease in not only heart-related events (such as heart attack and sudden death) but further revascularization procedures (such as angioplasty and bypass surgery) as compared to balloon angioplasty.

Like the AVERT Trial, the RITA 2 Trial punched holes in the belief that opening a blocked coronary artery with angioplasty improves the patient's prognosis. The results of this trial appeared in *the Journal of the American College of Cardiology* in 2003, and underscored the importance of conducting clinical trials to evaluate new forms of therapy. This trial found that balloon angioplasty did not reduce the risk of heart attack or death among study subjects—it actually increased it!

Stents

Interventional cardiologists were not about to give up without a fight. "Maybe balloon angioplasty alone doesn't improve the prognosis for the patient," they argued. "Stents work better." But when several clinical studies regarding the use of stents were finally presented at national cardiology meetings, it turned out that they, like coronary bypass surgery, didn't provide any benefit beyond that afforded by medical therapy alone. In fact, they often proved detrimental.

The first results presented were from the Occluded Artery Trial (OAT) at the annual meeting of the American Heart Association in November 2006. (The full results appeared in the influential *New England Journal of Medicine*, in 2007.) The study concluded that stent placement in the occluded artery responsible for the recent heart attack did *not* reduce the occurrence of death, and did *not* reduce the occurrence of repeat heart attack or heart failure. In fact, there was an *increase* in repeat heart attacks among patients receiving stents during the study's four years of follow-up. What seemed to make sense—opening a blocked artery with a stent following a heart attack—was conclusively found *not* to be beneficial, and in some respects even detrimental.

The Courage Trial, which was presented in New Orleans at a meeting of the American College of Cardiology in March 2007 and appeared in the *New England Journal of Medicine* shortly thereafter, found similar results. The seven-year study was designed to find out whether stents reduced the risk of heart attack or death in patients with coronary blockages who were already on maximum medical therapy. The study found no additional advantage to putting in a stent. (Courage, incidentally, was a good name for the study—it did indeed take courage on the part of the clinical investigators who conducted it, since many interventional cardiologists felt the researchers were putting patients with significant blockages in harm's way by denying them the "benefit" of stent insertion to "fix" the problem.)

Greek researchers D. G. Katritsis and colleagues performed a meta-analysis of multiple clinical trials in an effort to evaluate more broadly the merits of angioplasty and stent placement versus "conservative therapy" (meaning, in this case, medication). After objectively analyzing information drawn from eleven separate studies, they too concluded that coronary intervention did not offer any benefit in terms of long-term, hard clinical outcomes as compared with conservative medical treatment. As reported in the journal *Circulation* in 2005, they concluded that many surgical interventions in patients not in the midst of an acute cardiac event (such as a heart attack) "probably are not justified."

Most cardiologists assumed the problem with both angioplasty and stents was the gradual return of blockage to the cleared arteries. Roughly one-third of the patients who received stents had a return of their coronary blockage within six months. In an attempt to remedy this situation, companies developed coated stents. Unlike the original bare metal variation, these stents were covered in chemicals to make it less likely that coronary blockage would return. Millions of these new stents were inserted—again, without sufficient clinical study. And soon, it became apparent that coated stents could result in a catastrophic complication: sudden, unpredictable clotting that occurred at the stent site and led to heart attack or sudden cardiac death, especially in patients who either stopped or were taken off their blood thinners.

The Problem

How could all those doctors have been so wrong? All those cardiologists, with their catheters and their extensive medical training—how could they have been so far off base when it came to these procedures? It all goes back to that pipe metaphor.

Our cardiovascular system, you'll recall from chapter 2, doesn't work like household plumbing. Heart disease is not caused by a simple build-up of cholesterol inside the blood vessel; the process is more complex than that. LDL cholesterol enters the artery wall and gets oxidized, where it kicks off an inflammatory response that results in the formation of atheromatous plaques. These plaques can grow in size over time, in which case collateral vessels develop to compensate for the diminished blood flow. The real danger is that the plaques, re-gardless of size, may rupture and cause blood clots that can suddenly block the flow of blood through the artery, resulting in a heart attack or sudden cardiac death.

But many doctors are still treating arteries as if they were pipes. If the pipe metaphor were apt—if the threat were as sim-ple as built-up blockage, and the solution as simple as finding ways around or through that blockage—bypass surgery would work. Opening arteries with angioplasty and holding them open with stents would fix patients. But because our arteries aren't pipes, bypass surgery *doesn't* work. And angioplasty and stents *don't* fix patients.

The danger of heart disease lies in its unpredictability. Patients with heart disease don't just have a handful of large plaques that make themselves clearly known through symptoms like chest pain. Patients with heart disease can have dozens or even hun-dreds of plaques. If we could insert a stent or create a bypass in the case of every single one of those plaques, maybe surgical intervention would work. But the idea is absurd. Surgery that extensive would be even more dangerous than current bypass surgery—and most plaques are too small to see even with im-aging scans. So which blockage do you bypass? Where do you put the stent? Deciding is like throwing darts while blindfold-ed; your chances of picking the right plaque, like your chances of hitting a bull's-eye, are very, very low.

Intervention doesn't work because you can't be sure you'll get every single plaque, and even if you could, unless you ad-dress the underlying causes of plaque formation, more will de-velop. The only solution for heart disease is to work to prevent existing plaques from rupturing, and to prevent new plaques from forming in the first place.

Metabolic, Not Surgical

Neither plaque formation nor plaque rupture is simple or straightforward. They both occur because of complex interactions between cholesterol, free radicals, and inflammatory cells. All of these are controlled, either directly or indirectly, by our metabolic processes, which makes heart disease a metabolic disorder—a disorder caused by abnormal chemical reactions in the body that disrupt the normal process of metabolism (how we create energy from the food we eat). And metabolic disorders require metabolic solutions—not surgical ones.

Again, I'm not against surgery in *specific circumstances*—during heart attack, for example, when using a stent to open an artery or a bypass to restore blood flow may very well save heart muscle, and the patient's life. Or when patients continue to experience disabling chest pain despite maximal medical therapy, or have a critical blockage of the left main coronary artery. But surgery, in any circumstance, is like putting on a Band-Aid: it doesn't fix the problem; it just covers it up for a while.

If we want to stop heart disease, we have to address the underlying causes: cholesterol levels, free radical production, inflammation. The good news is that, because heart disease is a metabolic disorder, all of these things are, to a certain degree, *within our control*. No one has to die prematurely from heart disease. We have the knowledge, right now, to prevent and reverse the leading killer in America—without surgery,

Our bodies are affected not only by our genes, but by how we choose to live. Thanks to scientific advances in areas like transportation and food science over the last ten, fifty, even 2000 years, we've radically altered the way we live, from the foods we eat to how often we work up a sweat. But our bodies weren't designed to eat French fries and Twinkies or sit at desks for eight hours a day. And the result is metabolic havoc.

Preventing heart disease is in large part a matter of simply encouraging a healthy metabolism: eating the right foods, getting plenty of exercise, and avoiding chronic stress. And you can reverse heart disease the same way. Studies have shown this again and again, including one study published by Harvard-based researchers in the *New England Journal of Medicine* that concluded that lifestyle changes (diet, exercise, etc.) are capable of reducing cardiovascular disease risk by more than 80 percent—a figure which trumps even *statin drugs,* known to reduce the relative risk of cardiovascular disease risk by 30 to 35 percent. Heart disease symptoms are equally affected; the Lifestyle Heart Trial conducted by Dr. Dean Ornish found a 91 percent reduction in the frequency of chest pain through lifestyle changes alone. We'll look at a number of these studies (and more on how to prevent heart disease) in Part II.

But if all this is the case—and I can tell you from experience that it is—why aren't your doctors telling you this? Why does the treatment of heart disease still rely so thoroughly on surgery, which often doesn't work?

Why We Use Surgery Anyway

Surgical intervention is expensive, invasive, and carries significant risks. Even worse, large, well-designed clinical trials have repeatedly concluded that in the vast majority of patients there is simply *no evidence* that bypass surgeries or stent placements prevent heart attacks or prolong life. These facts have been published in black and white, for anyone to see, for decades. Yet cardiovascular intervention today is a multibillion-dollar industry. There are approximately one million angioplasties (mostly stent placements) and nearly a half million heart bypass operations performed each year in America. And the number of procedures is growing! How is it possible that doctors still regularly recommend surgery, promising it will "fix" their patients, in the face of so much evidence to the contrary? Who or what is to blame?

Eugene Braunwald, MD, professor emeritus at Harvard Medical School, authored an editorial published in 1977 in the prestigious *New England Journal of Medicine* that points to the answer. "An even more insidious problem is that an industry is being built around heart bypass surgery," wrote Dr. Braunwald. "This rapidly growing enterprise is developing a momentum of its own, and as time passes it will be progressively more difficult to curtail it if the results of carefully designed studies prove this step to be necessary."

Subsequent clinical trials did in fact clearly demonstrate that expensive coronary intervention procedures, by and large, are not medically warranted. And, as Braunwald feared, the industry's momentum has just as clearly rendered these procedures virtually impossible to stop. I can only speculate that Western medicine's emphasis on interventional treatment rather than preventive care, and the momentum that has built up around it, has created blinders that are hindering a majority of physicians from seeing the bigger picture.

Money almost certainly plays a role. While we might expect the medical profession to police itself and focus solely on what's proven to be best for the patient, tens of billions of dollars can have a way of making that focus go a little blurry. But money isn't the sole reason.

Heart surgery isn't always detrimental. In some cases, it's clearly beneficial, as in cardiac emergencies. And it's easy to understand how quantity could become linked to quality: if one heart surgery is good, 100 must be better, and 100,000 better still. As well, no hospital wants to be seen as doing the bare minimum of procedures.

Additionally, the current medical-legal climate may be playing a role. The threat of medical malpractice looms over virtually every decision physicians make these days, and I wouldn't be the first to suggest that the constant fear of being sued, and the exorbitant cost of medical malpractice insurance, is exerting undue influence on the practice of medicine in America. Some physicians respond to these pressures by leaving the field of medicine altogether. Others take an overly aggressive, cover-your-assets approach to virtually every case. It's quite possible that some physicians cling to the notion that doing something active, such as performing invasive procedures, is likely to be perceived as more proactive than simply sending a patient home with recommendations for medical therapy and lifestyle changes. Some doctors may simply feel they will find themselves in a more legally defensible position, should something go wrong, if they're able to say, "I performed state-of-the-art surgery to bypass the blockage . . . what more could I have done?"

Similarly, a cowboy mentality may come into play. After all, there's a certain fondness in America for taking action, any action, when confronted with a problem—never mind that the action in question may be the wrong one.

Whatever the reasons, the result is an industry that is like a runaway train—it is out of control.

Prevention, Not Intervention

The treatment of heart disease today—the cardiac intervention industry's reliance on surgery and disregard of lifestyle change—is a hoax of epic proportions. Its focus on intervention over prevention costs money, and it costs lives.

Our current approach to heart disease treatment is like an immense tower built on a shaky foundation. The cracks have begun to appear, and they're getting harder to ignore. But rather than rebuild on firm new ground, as the crumbling continues the cardiology juggernaut simply plasters over the growing cracks, and continues to add floors to the groaning edifice. The American cardiology empire is built upon the shaky foundation of too much heart surgery. But no one is willing to admit it.

Preventing heart disease by reversing the very process that

leads to heart attacks in the first place has always made more sense to me than attempting to patch up the coronary artery with a stent or bypass. In a way surgery is like patching a pothole-filled stretch of road. As anyone who lives in the northern United States knows, municipalities spend millions of dollars every winter filling in potholes with temporary patches. But the potholes just keep reappearing. Eventually, the municipality will be forced to either close the road or finally bite the bullet and completely resurface it, putting an end to constantly developing new potholes, and saving money (and automobile suspensions) in the long run.

In the first scenario, a temporary solution (pothole patches) is applied again and again at considerable expense, while the underlying problem (a crumbling road surface) is never addressed. Modern medicine's approach to the treatment of heart disease is much the same. Interventions like angioplasty and bypass surgery are temporary, expensive solutions to an underlying problem: an ongoing metabolic process of atherosclerosis that remains untouched by these quick "fixes."

Although surgical intervention has failed to fix or reverse coronary heart disease, we've made tremendous strides in our understanding of how atherosclerosis works, and how best to prevent and treat it metabolically. Part II gives you ten steps that will help you prevent, halt, and even reverse the progression of heart disease. It's an effective prevention program, which I've used successfully with my own patients for over twenty-five years, that helps ensure you and your family remain heart-healthy for a lifetime—no surgery needed!

CHAPTER 5

Pharmaceutical Follies

BEFORE WE TALK ABOUT how to prevent and reverse heart disease without surgery, it's worthwhile to take a quick detour through a few other things to be wary of in heart disease treatment. It's not just surgery that can be dangerous; the industry that's built up around our reliance on heart surgery has led to other practices that don't always have the best interests of the patient at heart. This chapter and the one that follows each look at an area where caution is recommended, beginning with prescription medication.

We live in an age of pharmaceutical wonders. Today, we have a pill for everything from infection to depression, from feeling a little sleepy to not feeling sleepy at all. In treating heart disease patients, too, our first line of defense is usually medication: to lower cholesterol, to prevent clots, to stabilize blood vessels, to minimize chest pain. And absolutely, these drugs work. So what's the problem?

The problem is not with the medications themselves so much as how they're used, and companies that sell them. But first, let's start by taking a look at the most frequently prescribed medications for various heart disease risk factors, and what exactly they do.

Heart Disease Medications

Foremost among heart disease medications are statins, cholesterol-lowering drugs developed in the 1980s. Statins were the first medication we could definitively say, through clinical trials, reduced the risk of dying from cardiovascular disease. Today, modern statins are, in most doctors' eyes, the first line of defense against atherosclerosis. Formally known as HMG-CoA reductase inhibitors, statins most popularly go by the brand names Crestor®, Zocor®, and Lipitor®, though generic statins are now available at significantly reduced cost. All act by inhibiting a crucial enzyme (HMG-CoA reductase) needed for cholesterol production within the body, and lower "bad" LDL cholesterol, through we've learned since that they may also work by decreasing the inflammation that leads to atheromatous plaques.

As with any drugs, statins can have serious side effects: muscle toxicity with secondary kidney failure and liver toxicity, among others. It is quite possible that these side effects are related to an unintended consequence of inhibiting HMG-CoA reductase. While HMG-CoA reductase is primarily used for cholesterol production, it's also needed for the production of something called Coenzyme Q10 (CoQ10), and statins' unintended reduction in CoQ10 production may contribute to muscle toxicity. Some scientists have recommended that anyone taking statin drugs should also take supplemental CoQ10.

The B vitamin niacin has been used for decades to lower "bad" LDL cholesterol, raise "good" HDL cholesterol, and lower triglycerides. Niacin also increases the size of cholesterol particles, making them less likely to enter the artery wall and become oxidized. However, its side effects, including flushing of the skin, have limited its use. More recently a long-acting form of niacin has been introduced, which appears to be better tolerated and more effective compared to traditional, short-acting niacin.

Fibrates are used to lower triglycerides and raise "good" HDL cholesterol. They work by decreasing the release of triglyceride-rich VLDL from the liver, increasing the activity of lipoprotein lipase activity, which in turn lowers triglyceride levels and increases levels of HDL cholesterol.

Resins, or bile acid sequestrants, were some of the first prescription medications used to reduce cholesterol. These agents bind bile acids in the gastrointestinal tract, decreasing the pool of bile acid in the liver. The liver then uses cholesterol to manufacture more bile acids, thereby decreasing the body's cholesterol levels. The problem with resins is that some patients find their side effects, including constipation, hard to live with. More recently, however, new, easier to tolerate versions have been introduced. One of the most recent, colesevelam, has also been shown to lower blood sugar levels in type-2 diabetes.

Cholesterol absorption inhibitors work by interfering with the absorption of cholesterol in the gastrointestinal tract. This medication can be taken by itself or it may be combined with statin medications for even more effective cholesterol-lowering (though clinical trials are still in progress to determine whether it truly reduces the risk of heart attack, stroke, and death when combined with a statin).

ACE inhibitors are used to lower blood pressure by decreasing the production of angiotensin 2, a protein that leads to the constriction of blood vessels and other adverse effects that result in an increase in blood pressure. ACE inhibitors have proven effective at decreasing heart attack risk among patients with cardiovascular disease risk factors. These drugs tend to be well tolerated, though some patients may develop a dry cough.

ARBs (angiotensin receptor blockers) also help to lower blood pressure by blocking angiotensin 2 at the receptor level, thus reducing the risk of cardiovascular events. Unlike ACE inhibitors, they seldom cause a cough.

Calcium channel blockers lower blood pressure by dilating blood vessels. They are also used to treat coronary artery spasm.

Medications Frequently Prescribed for Atherosclerosis		
Medication (generic/brand name)	What It Does	How It Works
Statins, or HMG-CoA reductase inhibitors		
simvastin/Zocor®, atorvastatin/Lipitor®, rosuvastatin/Crestor®, lovastatin/ Mevacor®	Reduces cholesterol levels	By decreasing the production of cholesterol in the body
Niacin		
niacin, long-acting niacin/Niaspan®	Lowers LDL cholesterol, raises HDL cholesterol, lowers triglycerides, lowers lipoprotein(a), and increases the size of cholesterol particles	By decreasing the production of triglyceride-rich VLDL in the liver and increasing triglyceride removal from the bloodstream
Fibrates		
fenofibrate/Tricor®, gemfibrozil/Lopid®	Lowers triglycerides and raises HDL cholesterol	By decreasing the release of triglyceride-rich VLDL from the liver and increasing triglyceride removal from the bloodstream
Resins, or bile acid sequestrants		
colesevelam/Welchol®	Lowers cholesterol	By binding to bile acids, making them inactive and thus forcing the liver to use cholesterol to manufacture more
Cholesterol absorption inhibitors		
ezetimibe/Zetia®	Lowers cholesterol	By partially blocking cholesterol absorption in the small bowel

ramipril/Altace®, lisinopril/Prinivil®	Lowers blood pressure	By decreasing the production of blood pressure–raising angiotensin 2
ARBs		
losartin/Cozaar®, valsartin/Diovan®, olmesartin/Benicar®	Lowers blood pressure	By blocking the effects of blood pressure–raising angiotensin 2
Calcium channel blockers		
amlodipine/Norvasc®	Lowers blood pressure, prevents blood-vessel spasm	By dilating blood vessels
Beta-blockers		
metaprolol/Toprol XL®, atenolol/Tenormin®, propranolol/Inderal®	Lowers blood pressure and heart rate	By blocking adrenaline
Nitroglycerine		
	Reduces chest pain	By dilating coronary arteries
Aspirin		
	Prevents blood clots and reduces inflammation	By blocking the effects of platelets and reducing inflammation

Beta blockers act by blocking natural hormones, like adrenaline, that mediate the "fight or flight" response in our body. These hormones work by binding with receptors on target organs, including the heart, which is richly studded with these receptors. Beta blockers bind to these receptors first, blocking the hormones' access and thus preventing them from raising heart rate and blood pressure. In addition, beta blockers are useful in treating heart rhythm disorders and congestive heart failure.

Nitroglycerine (NTG) has been used for over a century to treat chest pain, and can be given under the tongue, as an ointment applied to the skin, as a patch, or as a tablet or capsule. It works by dilating the coronary arteries, thereby improving blood flow to the heart.

Aspirin decreases the risk of heart attack and stroke by blocking the effects of platelets, the cells that contribute to clot formation. Aspirin may also lower cardiovascular risk by decreasing inflammation. Unless the patient has a contraindication to the use of aspirin (such as an aspirin allergy or a bleeding ulcer), most physicians advise all patients with cardiovascular disease to take aspirin on a regular basis. Note: Low-dose aspirin appears to be just as effective as high-dose aspirin for cardiovascular protection.

Many other medications are used in cardiovascular disease prevention, and new medications are constantly being developed—including genetically engineered "good" HDL cholesterol in pill form that could help reverse coronary artery disease by preventing cholesterol from remaining in the artery wall where it would lead to plaque development. As well, combination drug therapy, in which several different medications are combined into a single pill for enhanced efficacy, lower cost, and increased patient compliance with prescribed treatment, has lately gained in popularity.

Pharmaceutical Pitfalls

My biggest issue with heart disease medication is the belief that using them releases us from the responsibility of living a healthy lifestyle. Instead of using medications to *augment* responsible behavior, we use them to excuse ourselves from it: "I'm on Lipitor so I can eat whatever I want," a patient once told me after his discharge from the hospital following heart bypass surgery.

But my second biggest issue is with the pharmaceutical industry. Pharmaceutical companies spend millions of dollars a year on research and development and product testing—and that's a good thing. The discovery of penicillin changed the world. The development of statins has certainly changed the way we treat heart disease. My issue with the pharmaceutical industry isn't with what they do, just the way they do it.

I'm actually a big believer in medications—when they're used to reinforce lifestyle changes, not when they're used in place of them. The pharmaceutical industry would have us believe a pill is the solution to any condition we may have. And convincing us of this keeps them in business, even when our health might be better served in other ways.

Medications are also far more expensive than they need to be. The difference in cost between prescriptions here and just over the border in Canada is staggering—even after factoring in socialized health care. But the biggest hoax here has to do with brand name medications and their generic counterparts.

When a company develops a new medication, they patent it, which means only they can sell that particular combination of chemicals. But that patent is only good for a defined period of time. After that point, the drug can be duplicated and sold under a different name. These similar, cheaper "generic" drugs do the same thing as their brand name counterparts, and are usually just as effective; they're just less expensive, which cuts into pharmaceutical companies' profits.

Pharmaceutical companies fight tooth and nail to keep new drugs under patent for as long as they can, and are sometimes able to delay generics from coming to market for years. Alternately, they may tinker with the original drug formula enough to make the drug qualify as "new" under patent law without actually affecting the efficacy—and then claim it works *better* than the old drug's newly released generic in order to keep their customers from switching. As a result, many people are putting themselves into debt in order to afford these more expensive—but not necessarily more effective—medications, when they could buy the generic for as low as $4 at Wal-Mart.

Another way pharmaceutical companies convince consumers to pay more than they need to is through direct-to-consumer marketing, and through marketing to physicians. Effective advertising can gain companies a larger share of consumer dollars unrelated to their products' medical benefits. And doctors are supplied with everything from free sample pills to free lunches and other perks so that they might choose one company's drug over another. Pharmaceutical companies can also reward doctors according to their prescribing practices; the companies have easy access to records of exactly who has been prescribing their pills, or what they're prescribing instead. The decision as to what medication to prescribe a patient can end up having less to do with what would be the best, most cost-effective medication, and more to do with who has the most effective advertisements and sales force.

What You Can Do

The solution here is to make sure you're educated. Ask your doctor if a less expensive generic version of the brand name medication prescribed would be just as effective. And remember: medication is never a substitute for a healthy lifestyle. Diet and exercise is often the most effective way to lower cholesterol, blood sugar, and blood pressure.

CHAPTER 6

The Radiation Ruse
Beware of Unnecessary CAT Scans and Nuclear Stress Tests

There is no safe level of radiation exposure and there is no dose of radiation so low that the risk of a malignancy is zero.
—Dr. Karl Z. Morgan, the "Father of Health Physics"

IN MEDICINE, WE ARE TAUGHT to use something called the "risk-benefit ratio," which guides us in deciding what treatment is appropriate for each individual patient in each situation. Cases like those in an emergency room, where a patient has obvious, life-threatening symptoms, require doctors to find out what's going on as quickly and accurately as possible in order to select the most appropriate treatment, even if the method of diagnosis carries risk. The benefits of having the diagnosis quickly—the patient not dying—outweigh the risks in achieving it—for example, the risk associated with exploratory surgery. In cases where the threat of death is not so imminent, the process of diagnosis is different. If you can effectively diagnose the patient using other, less risky methods, those methods should be exhausted first.

Most uses of the risk-benefit ratio in medicine are less clear-cut than that, of course. But one area where the risks and benefits are often not weighted as clearly as they ought to be is medical imaging. In cardiac medicine, there are two imaging tests that deliver significant radiation exposure and are frequently used unnecessarily: the CAT scan, and the nuclear stress test.

The CAT Scam

When cardiac CAT scans are used during an emergency situation, they can provide critical diagnostic information about coronary blood flow that can help save a patient's life. This is where this technology shines.

The problem is that too many health care professionals casually recommend these scans to patients who are healthy, have no symptoms, and just want to know what's going on inside their bodies. These machines expose the patient to an astounding amount of radiation, often the equivalent of up to 750 chest X-rays. This radiation exposure can often lead to strand breaks in DNA that result in mutations linked to the initiation of cancer. The medical profession may thus be on the verge of creating a dramatic increase in the number of cancer cases. In addition, due to aggressive marketing, CAT scans are now used indiscriminately in many offices, clinics, walk-in centers, and hospitals throughout the country. You don't even need a doctor's prescription to have one done.

For many years, I have been concerned about the dramatic increase in radiation exposure due to diagnostic testing performed by radiologists and cardiologists. Recently, the *New England Journal of Medicine* reported on this growing danger. Currently, the authors suggest that over 20 million adults are being exposed to potentially unnecessary radiation. The article reaches the same conclusion that I have been speaking about for years: we need to urgently reduce the number of questionable CAT scans in order to dramatically reduce our risk of cancer.

What Is the CAT Scan?

Invented in 1972 by Godfrey Hounsfield and Allan Cormack, who later won a Nobel Prize, CAT (computerized axial tomographic) or CT scans use both X-rays and computer technology to create detailed images of body parts, including the heart and other organs, bones, and muscles. Unlike traditional X-rays, the CAT scan X-ray beam moves around, creating many different views, or "slices," of its intended subject. A computer is then used to combine these picture slices into highly detailed three-dimensional images that are useful in helping physicians clearly visualize and diagnose disorders.

Before CAT scans became widely available, the cardiologist's primary diagnostic tool was the angiogram, or heart catheterization, an invasive procedure requiring hospitalization and carrying serious risks. So when the first CAT scans appeared on the scene, they seemed like a great advancement. The recently developed 64-slice CAT scan is even more impressive: it takes thousands of images of the heart in just a few seconds, allowing a cardiologist to see exactly how a patient's heart is functioning. Today patients can to walk into a scanning center and leave less than an hour later with a complete, detailed picture of their heart or even their whole body. Soon, the 128-slice CAT scan will be widely available, and even more precise machines are in the works. The scans are available without a doctor's prescription and have been heavily promoted through media advertising, endorsements by prominent physicians, and even television celebrities. A *Time* magazine cover story in 2005 summed it up: "How New Heart-Scanning Technology Could Save Your Life." The rush was on for everyone to get 64-slice whole-body scans—even on an annual basis—to make sure nothing was wrong with them or to catch anything that was wrong in its early, treatable stages.

As a preventive cardiologist first hearing about the CAT scan, I thought it sounded close to miraculous: a simple, noninvasive, painless test that quickly provided a highly detailed picture of the heart, giving us the ability to pinpoint coronary blockages and other early signs of disease so we could treat them before any further damage occurred. Or better yet, the scan might find nothing wrong with the heart at all, allowing us to reassure patients and let them go on with their lives.

However, it hasn't quite turned out that way. It is now apparent that CAT scans present many significant risks, especially when used for screening patients with no symptoms of disease. Too many people, including health care professionals, are not aware of these risks and, as a result, may be unnecessarily endangering their patients' health and even lives.

Cat Scan Concerns

Before discussing the risks posed by CAT scans, we must make a distinction between the two uses of these devices: scanning and diagnosis. *My objections are solely to the use of CAT scans for screening people who have no symptoms* and just want to find out what's going on inside their bodies, whether due to their own curiosity or a recommendation by health care professionals.

I have no problem with CAT scans for patients who truly need these tests, such as those who show up in the emergency room with crushing chest pains. Using a 64-slice CAT scanner and other imaging modalities can help us make a very rapid diagnosis of whether or not these patients have blockages in their arteries causing a heart attack, or blood clots in their lungs, or dissections of their arteries. In situations like these, CAT scans can unquestionably be lifesavers. The benefits of getting information from a CAT scan in such circumstances are clearly outweighed by the risk to the patient.

THE PRIMARY DANGERS OF CONVENTIONAL CARDIAC CAT SCANS
My major concerns about cardiac CAT scans are as follows:
1. Excess exposure to radiation.
2. Cost to patient (and the excessive profit obtained by the health care industry).
3. Lack of proven effectiveness.
4. Potential for additional tests and procedures that are costly, could have adverse health consequences, and are often unnecessary.
5. Use of scans to "motivate patients," which could be better accomplished by talking to and educating patients about lifestyle changes.
6. Ready availability of safe, effective methods that accomplish the same goals.

The Dangers of Radiation

The most serious problem with the widespread use of CAT scans is the radiation these devices leave in our bodies. CAT scans are not simple chest X-rays, which deliver only a small amount of radiation. Instead, they expose the patient to a significant amount of radiation, and radiation in significant doses has been shown to increase the risk of cancer.

We are all exposed to "natural background radiation"—that is, radiation from the sun, radon gas, rocks in the ground, cosmic rays, and other sources that usually can't be avoided in our daily lives. Radiation is measured in units called "millisieverts" (mSv), and we can use millisieverts to compare this natural radiation to the levels of radiation we get from other sources, such as medical tests. For instance, a chest X-ray provides about 0.02 mSv, or the equivalent of 2.4 days of natural background radiation. A CAT scan of the abdomen, on the other hand, provides about 10.0 mSv, or the equivalent of 500 chest X-rays or 3.3 *years* of natural background radiation. And a 64-slice whole-body CAT scan provides 15.2 mSv for men and 21.4 mSv for women (women's denser body tissue and breasts require higher doses to get clear images)—quite a difference, especially when you realize that the radiation you receive is cumulative.

Now compare these numbers with the level of radiation to which Japanese survivors of the atomic bomb explosions at Hiroshima and Nagasaki were exposed: an average dose of between 5 and 20 mSv, with some doses as high as 50 mSv. A single CAT scan can easily exceed that average. And since radiation from all sources remains in our bodies for life, the likelihood of the average twenty-first-century patient matching or exceeding that average, even without a CAT scan, is very high. In the *New York Times*, Roni Caryn Rabin reported that recent studies indicate that the amount of radiation in the bodies of Americans increased 600 percent between 1980 and 2006, with the bulk of this increase attributed to diagnostic imaging procedures. In 1980 about 3 million of these procedures were performed, but by 2006 the number had skyrocketed to 62 million. If you were to follow some popular recommendations to have an annual CAT scan, plus one virtual colonoscopy and a coronary angiogram (both of which also deliver large doses of radiation), in the space of only a few years you could easily be exposed to more radiation than even the most highly exposed Hiroshima survivor.

The World Health Organization, Centers for Disease Control and Prevention, and the National Institute of Environmental Health Sciences have all classified X-rays as carcinogens based on the fact that they have been linked to leukemia and cancers of the breast, lungs, and thyroid. The risk of a fatal cancer from a chest X-ray has been estimated as one in a million or more—in other words, very remote. But the risk of a fatal cancer in a person who has had just one of these new 64-slice CAT scans is estimated to be one in 2,000. In one study reported in the *Journal of the American Medical Association*, the risk of cancer in people having 64-slice CAT scans of the heart was found to be greater for young women than young men. Researchers found that one of every 143 women scanned at age twenty will develop cancer, usually breast cancer; the risk for forty-year-old

> ## "SUPER X-RAYS" SET THE STAGE FOR FUTURE CANCER
>
> The average American's radiation exposure has increased dramatically since 1980, largely due to increases in the use of computerized axial tomography (CAT or CT) scans. These "super X-rays" deliver far more radiation than conventional plain-film X-rays, which are already classified as carcinogens by the World Health Organization and the federal Centers for Disease Control and Prevention.
>
> Use of CAT scans has increased by more than a factor of twenty since 1980. While CAT scans have revolutionized diagnostic radiology, and immediate patient benefit/risk ratios are favorable, a new study published in the *New England Journal of Medicine* concludes that increased radiation exposure is setting the stage for future cancer cases.
>
> "There is a strong case to be made that too many C[A]T studies are being performed in the United States," write the study's authors. The greatest increases have been in diagnostic procedures in children (particularly in the diagnosis of appendicitis) and in elective screening procedures in adults (such as full-body scans and virtual colonoscopies). Children's CAT scans are especially troubling, as children are more susceptible to the damaging effects of ionizing radiation than adults. "Perhaps 20 million adults and, crucially, more than 1 million children per year in the United States are being irradiated unnecessarily."

women falls to one in 284. For men, the cancer risk was one in 686 for a twenty-year-old, and one in 1,007 for a forty-year-old. The reason for the gender difference in risk lies in the fact that breast tissue is very sensitive to radiation and the heart can't be scanned without radiation exposure to breast tissue. Clearly, administering CAT scans simply for screening is a risk we shouldn't be recommending people take.

There is no level of radiation exposure below which you can assume you're safe. Of course, everyone is different and no one will be affected by radiation in the same way. And when we talk about the radiation doses for various medical procedures, we are always talking about estimates rather than exact figures. Depending on where you have your CAT scan done, who is performing it, what machine is being used, and what condition is being screened for, the doses can vary. But radiation interferes with the body's natural immune system the same way regardless of dose. Your body keeps you healthy by attacking free radicals, scavengers, and cancer cells inside you, but its resources are finite. A sudden blast of radiation can be just the impetus needed to allow leukemia, breast cancer, or some other cancer to begin developing.

Cost

When CAT scan machines were first widely introduced in the early 1980s, they were heavily publicized and marketed. Because the scans were normally not covered by insurance, the cost was all out-of-pocket for the patient. So a lot of people, especially those who had cause to be worried about potential health risks due to family history, put thousands of dollars on the table—even if they couldn't afford it—all because they and their families believed the tests would "save their lives" by revealing hidden life-threatening conditions. Some of my own patients told me that imaging centers had charged them up to $2,500 for a single scan; other patients have reported paying anywhere from $500 to $5,000. And many of these centers were not run by doctors but by business people who were very aggressive in their marketing.

Hospitals, doctors, and scanning centers had invested several million dollars in each one of these scanners, and naturally they wanted to recoup their costs. So there was a lot of pressure put on patients to have CAT scans when they may not have needed them and a lot of marketing done to doctors about how they could double their income by using these machines in their practices. The dangers were being completely ignored. Unfortunately, this is still largely the case.

Effectiveness

Here's what most people do not realize: there is absolutely no data to prove that CAT scans are medically useful for people who do not have any symptoms. According to the FDA website:

> The FDA has never approved CT for screening any part of the body for any specific disease, let alone for screening the whole body

when there are no specific symptoms of disease at all. No manufacturer has submitted data to FDA to support the safety and efficacy of screening claims for whole-body CT screening.

They further state:

the FDA knows of no data demonstrating that whole-body CT screening is effective in detecting any particular disease early enough for the disease to be managed, treated, or cured and advantageously spare a person at least some of the detriment associated with serious illness or premature death.

In addition, the American College of Radiology, the American College of Cardiology/American Heart Association, the American Association of Physicists in Medicine, and the American Medical Association, among others, do not recommend CAT scans. Medicare and most insurance companies do not cover CAT scans for screening because the tests have never been shown to provide information in addition to what we can already learn through doing a medical history, a physical exam, and blood tests.

What to Do with the Results

COMPARISON OF RADIATION DOSES			
Procedure	Typical effective dose (mSv)	No. of chest X-rays for equivalent effective dose	Time for equivalent effective dose from natural background radiation
Chest X-ray	0.02	1	2.4 days
CAT head	2.0	100	243 days
CAT abdomen	10.0	500	3.3 years
Coronary angiogram	3.4	170	1.1 years
64-slice CAT (male)	15.2	760	5.1 years
64-slice CAT (female)	21.4	1070	7.1 years

Apart from the serious radiation issue, the biggest problem with CAT scans is what to do with the results. Let's look at different scenarios, depending on whether the results are normal or abnormal.

If the results are normal: The patient is given a clean bill of health. The danger here is not immediate, but long-term. If the patient is living an unhealthy lifestyle, a normal test result may give him or her the excuse he or she needs to continue those habits—and end up suffering from disease later down the road. And that's the *best* case scenario. We also have to consider the possibility that the test results are a false negative, and the patient does actually have health problems, but they either did not show up on the test or were not correctly interpreted. In this case, the patient has received a hefty dose of radiation, has not gotten any useful results, and may delay coming in for a developing health problem in the future because he or she is confident in their results.

If the test results are abnormal: The test shows a blockage, and the doctor recommends further testing. The patient goes to an invasive cardiologist and gets a heart catheterization, which shows an 80 percent blockage, and the patient, who had no symptoms before the CAT scan, has a stent implanted to protect him or her from future heart attack. But as we learned in chapter 4, there is no evidence that subjecting asymptomatic individuals to stents or bypass surgery will reduce their subsequent risk of heart attack or prolong their lives. So not only has the patient's chances of having a heart attack not been decreased, in many respects it's actually been *increased*, since putting in a stent can trigger a sudden and catastrophic heart attack or even death. In any circumstance, a positive CAT scan is likely to result in additional costs, risks, and unnecessary procedures for the patient.

A Better Approach

For patients who have no symptoms, a far more effective approach to health is to sit down with their physician, and have them take a good history, see if there is a family history of heart disease, do a thorough examination, find out if the blood pressure is elevated, check the pulse, listen to the heart, do an EKG and blood tests, and then talk about how to follow a healthy lifestyle, if the individual is not already doing so.

In the event that you and your doctor agree that a CAT scan is a medical necessity after taking those steps, you should discuss whether there are any alternative tests, such as an MRI. MRI, or magnetic resonance imaging, uses magnetic fields to generate images, and unlike CAT scans, MRIs do not produce any radiation exposure.

The long-held belief that CAT scan results motivate people to change their lifestyles has been found to be untrue. A study in the *Journal of the American Medical Association* found that these scans did not change behavior in any way—abnormal scans simply did not motivate patients to change their lifestyles or take their medication any more regularly. Furthermore, is it really appropriate to subject patients to the risk and expense of CAT scans to "motivate" them to do what they should be doing anyway?

The word "doctor" means "teacher," and we doctors should be spending our time teaching patients how to live healthy lives, not ordering screening tests like CAT scans that have potential adverse consequences. Part of the problem is that when doctors do take the time to talk with patients and explain things to them carefully, they are not rewarded. I've been a preventive cardiologist for over two decades and have spent a lot of time with my patients teaching them how to stay healthy. You don't get paid for that, at least not in this country. In many other countries, such as Canada and France, doctors are paid for keeping their patients healthy, which seems like a far more effective approach to me than a health care system that rewards intervention over prevention. We need to get back to what we know works.

WHAT YOU NEED TO KNOW: AVOIDING THE RADIATION DANGERS OF CARDIAC CAT SCANS
• One of the most important advances in modern medicine was the development of computerized axial tomography (CAT or CT) scans.
• While they provide valuable information, CAT scans expose the body to a large amount of radiation, an amount far greater than earlier technologies like X-rays. Ionizing radiation produced by CAT scans is a known carcinogen even in lower doses.
• The annual number of CAT scans performed in the United States skyrocketed from 3 million scans in 1980 to an estimated 62 million scans today. Many scientists believe an epidemic of radiation-induced cancer is imminent.
• Radiation exposure is cumulative over the course of a lifetime, and it is particularly damaging when it occurs at a young age.
• With one or more CAT scans, it is possible to accrue the amount of radiation exposure experienced by survivors of Hiroshima and Nagasaki, who later succumbed to cancer.
• While CAT scans have an important role in diagnosing symptomatic patients, they should not be used as screening tools for healthy individuals. There are no demonstrated benefits of screening asymptomatic patients, while the risks of radiation exposure are well documented.
• In healthy patients, a better preventive health strategy involves regular check-ups, screening for cardiovascular risk factors such as blood lipids, and practicing a healthy lifestyle.

Nuclear Stress Testing

Cardiac stress tests evaluate how much oxygenated blood reaches the heart muscle during exercise compared to when the body is at rest. Abnormalities in the test indicate a blockage may be present in the coronary artery. To do the test, the patient is put on a treadmill and hooked up to an EKG. The patient's EKG pattern, blood pressure, and other symptoms are then checked regularly as the patient exercises.

The stress test can be an important tool for detecting serious blockages. However, stress testing only detects significant blockages (blockages of 75 percent or more) that reduce blood flow to the heart during exercise, and as we've learned, severe blockages are far less likely to cause heart attacks than small blockages, which stress tests don't detect.

The accuracy of a stress test in detecting coronary blockages can be improved by combining it with an imaging test. Two types of stress imaging tests are the nuclear stress test and the stress echo test. Both of these tests can improve the diagnostic accuracy of the stress test. In nuclear stress testing, however, a radioactive isotope is injected intravenously, delivering a significant amount of radiation. As we saw with the CAT scan, radiation never actually leaves your body; patients who go through nuclear stress tests remain "hot" for weeks afterward, even setting off airport radiation detectors. Contrast this with a stress echo test, which utilizes harmless sound waves instead of radioactive material to image the heart. The accuracy of a stress echo study is similar to a stress nuclear study and, in addition to being safe, is less expensive.

As with CAT scans, part of the danger of a stress test lies in what you do with the information obtained from it. A normal test result does not mean you are not at risk for a heart attack, and it isn't an excuse not to follow a heart-healthy lifestyle. Likewise, an abnormal test result doesn't mean the blockage found necessarily warrants surgery or angioplasty; it may be perfectly stable, and best treated with lifestyle changes and medical therapy.

The Take-Home Message

The take-home message is this: make sure you're able to make educated decisions about your treatment and testing. If your doctor recommends a CAT scan, ask if it is truly necessary and if there are alternative imaging tests that don't involve radiation exposure. If your doctor wants to do a nuclear stress test, ask if a stress echo study would suffice.

If you and your doctor do decide that performing a CAT scan or nuclear stress test is a medical necessity, find out how much radiation you'll be receiving—and keep track. It is important that you have a good idea of approximately how much radiation you are carrying around in your body and that you discuss this with your physician whenever any test involving radiation is recommended.

It would be great if every time a patient was given a test involving radiation, they were told of the risks and the amount of radiation involved, but that just isn't the case. Until it is, the burden is on the patient to protect him- or herself.

PART TWO

THE SOLUTION

The Ozner 10-Step
Prevention Program

S USAN, A SCHOOLTEACHER, suffered a very mild
heart attack about ten years ago. She underwent an angioplasty, but shortly thereafter experienced some mild
chest pain. So another angioplasty was performed.
And on it went; over the next few years Susan endured
six angioplasties. When the time came for the seventh, Susan
balked. "I'm a widow," she told me when she came to my office
looking for an alternative. "My husband died in a car accident
and I'm raising my twelve-year-old daughter." Her eyes filled
with tears as she continued. "These angioplasties are not doing
the job. I'm scared that I'm going to have a major heart attack
and die, and my daughter will be left all alone."

Another of my patients, Jack, first came to see me as a young
attorney. Like Susan, Jack was terrified. His father had suffered
a heart attack and had undergone coronary bypass surgery, but
had died on the operating table. "The doctors told me that I
have severe blockages in two of my coronary arteries," he explained. "They told me I'm a 'ticking time bomb' and if I don't
have surgery, I'll never live to see my kids grow up. When I
stormed out of the hospital," he continued, "they even made

me sign a statement saying I was leaving against medical advice, because I might collapse in the parking lot." He was clearly upset and understandably so, given his father's experience with bypass surgery. And he was anguished by his doctors' insistence that there were no viable alternatives to surgery. He had even found it difficult to find another physician willing to accept him as a patient, having evidently been blacklisted as a "noncompliant patient." "But Dr. Ozner," he said, "these are the exact same things they told my father. I just have a feeling that, if I go in for surgery, like him, I'll never come out."

Another patient of mine, Fred, was a prominent member of the community. Fred was often tired and sometimes short of breath, but he had no symptoms that indicated serious heart disease. A heart catheterization, performed several months ago at another institution, revealed a moderate blockage in one of his coronary arteries. I did not recommend stent insertion; rather, I told him I felt the best approach was a comprehensive prevention program. While I was out of town at a meeting a few months later, however, he saw another cardiologist who persuaded him to have a stent inserted.

If you picked up this book, it's likely that you or someone you care about either is at high risk for or has heart disease. You've had experiences like Jack's, Susan's, or Fred's. And you picked up this book hoping to educate yourself, and hoping to find a way of preventing or reversing heart disease. You picked up this book hoping to save your life, or the life of someone you love. And I'm about to show you how.

I can't guarantee you will live forever, any more than I can guarantee that you will avoid all disease. But I can say with certainty that, by following these ten steps, you *will* vastly improve your chances of preventing, and even reversing, heart disease. (Though it is recommended that you discuss all lifestyle changes and medical therapy with your physician. The optimal approach for preventing heart attack and stroke is a prevention strategy that is discussed between the patient and his or her treating physician!)

It is important to note that while following any of these steps will improve your health somewhat, it's only by following all of them that you gain the maximum benefit. All of these steps are intimately and inextricably connected. The first three steps outline lifestyle changes that have been proven to reduce your risk of heart disease. Steps 4 through 8 detail the specific metabolic processes most closely involved with heart disease, how the lifestyle changes in steps 1 through 3 affect them, and other ways to assist in their management. And steps 9 and 10 discuss how to best leverage modern medicine to diagnose and treat impairment in these metabolic processes and the heart disease that can result.

I put Susan on an earlier version of this prevention plan. And she's never had to have another heart catheterization or angioplasty. She had high LDL (bad) cholesterol and low HDL (good) cholesterol, factors that were never addressed by any of the procedures she'd undergone, and after following my prevention plan, her cholesterol levels have been normal for years. On her last visit, she came to my office smiling, with tears of joy in her eyes, as she showed me photographs of her daughter's wedding.

I did the same with Jack. He still refused to submit to surgery, but he followed my advice avidly. Nearly three decades later, he's still going strong. In fact, a few years ago he needed hip surgery and underwent a pre-operative cardiac catheterization. And guess what? The procedure revealed that the blockages he had when he first came to me—the blockages that were going to kill him before he could leave the hospital parking lot—had virtually disappeared.

And Fred? I would like to be able to tell you that everything turned out okay for Fred, but unfortunately, I can't. He never made it out of the operating room. During the angioplasty procedure, his coronary artery ruptured and he was hustled into the operating room for emergency surgery. He died on the table.

These ten steps are the very best advice I can give you for the prevention and treatment of heart disease. It's the advice I give to every patient I see in my cardiology practice, and it's advice I myself follow every day. But your health is in your hands, and no one else's. Taking the necessary steps to prevent or reverse heart disease is up to you.

STEP 1

Follow a Mediterranean Diet

Let food be your medicine.

—HIPPOCRATES

WHAT YOU EAT is the single most important factor in your health. It's something you have an incredible amount of control over (because you make decisions about it every day) and something that affects you at every level (because what you eat provides the building blocks for everything in your body). It plays a part, directly or indirectly, in every other prevention step that follows. And clinical studies have proved that the best way to eat, for heart disease prevention and for overall health and well-being, is a way that's been followed for over a thousand years: a Mediterranean diet.

The study that changed the way I think about the connection between diet and health was the Seven Countries Study, the twenty-year study I described back in chapter 1 that showed that men living in the Mediterranean region had the lowest incidence of heart disease and the longest life expectancy. This study prompted the lead author, Dr. Ancel Keys, to ask, "If some developed countries can do without heart attacks, why can't we?" But the Seven Countries Study is far from the only study that demonstrated the benefits of a Mediterranean diet. A brief summary of a few of the most important:

THE LYON DIET HEART STUDY

This study compared a Mediterranean diet to a control diet resembling the American Heart Association Step 1 diet in heart attack survivors. It found that, compared to the American Heart Association Step 1 diet, the Mediterranean diet afforded significantly better protection against recurrent heart attack and death. The Mediterranean diet was associated with a 70 percent decrease in risk of death and a 73 percent decrease in risk of recurrent cardiac events.

THE SINGH INDO-MEDITERRANEAN DIET STUDY

This study placed 499 patients with risk factors for coronary heart disease on an Indo-Mediterranean diet. It found that the diet change resulted in a reduction in serum cholesterol and was associated with a significant reduction in heart attack and sudden cardiac death. Subjects were also found to have fewer cardiovascular events than those on a conventional diet.

THE ALZHEIMER'S DISEASE STUDY

This study by Dr. Nikolaos Scarmeas and colleagues from Columbia University Medical Center in New York demonstrated that a Mediterranean diet reduced the risk of developing Alzheimer's disease by 68 percent. Another study from this same group showed that patients with Alzheimer's disease who followed a Mediterranean diet had reduced mortality.

THE METABOLIC SYNDROME STUDY

This study by Dr. Katherine Esposito and colleagues from Italy evaluated the effects of a Mediterranean diet on patients with metabolic syndrome (obesity, elevated blood sugar, elevated blood pressure, abnormal cholesterol profile, and markers of vascular inflammation; see step 8). A Mediterranean diet was shown to improve all of the components of metabolic syndrome.

The results of these studies are clear. But why is a Mediterranean diet so much more effective in preventing heart disease and other illness?

The Toxic American Diet

Our toxic American diet is killing us. Part of the reason is what our typical American diet doesn't include: enough fresh fruit and vegetables, or whole grains, for example. Many processed foods widely available in our supermarkets and fast-food outlets have been effectively stripped of their key healthful ingredients. But most of the reason is what our diet *does* include. Our food is contaminated with pesticides and artificial preservatives, and contains an excessive amount of unhealthy fats, high fructose corn syrup, and sodium. Let's take a look at a couple of these, and their negative health effects, in-depth.

Unhealthy Fats

There are three types of fat in our diet: unsaturated fat, saturated fat, and trans fat. Unsaturated fats, including polyunsaturated fats and monounsaturated fats, are healthy fats. Polyunsaturated fats include omega-3 and omega-6 fatty acids. Omega-3, which comes from oily fish, vegetables, and nuts, decreases the risk of heart disease. Monounsaturated fat, from nuts, seeds, and olive oil, has a positive impact on our cholesterol ratio and helps to decrease inflammation. Vegetable oils (which include various amounts of both mono- and polyunsaturated fats) like soybean, sunflower, and corn oils, are neutral, meaning they have no effect, either good or bad, on heart health.

Saturated fats, which raise "bad" LDL cholesterol and increase the risk of heart disease and cancer, are unhealthy fats. They're found in animal products, such as red meat, butter, milk, cheese, and lard, as well as tropical oils, like coconut and palm oils.

Then there are trans fatty acids, or trans fats. Trans fats don't occur naturally; they're manufactured by taking oils—mainly vegetable oils—and putting them through a process called hydrogenation. Trans fats are found in foods such as margarine, French fries, potato chips, cookies, crackers, baked goods, and frozen foods, and were developed so that foods could last longer on the shelf without becoming rancid.

These fats are particularly harmful to our health, as they raise "bad" LDL cholesterol, lower "good" HDL cholesterol, increase inflammation, and make blood clots more likely to form. Trans fat consumption has been linked to heart disease, cancer, and diabetes. Trans fat can be so harmful that certain countries have even banned them from their food supply. Until America does the same, the best course of action is to pay attention to nutrition labels, avoid food that contains trans fat or partially hydrogenated oil, and limit our consumption of saturated fat.

Beware of the trans fat hoax: Food companies are allowed to list zero trans fat on their label and still have up to 500 mg of trans fat per serving. This can result in a significant amount of trans fat consumption per day by duped consumers who think they are eating healthy. Since our own government doesn't protect us, we have to protect ourselves. If the nutritional label lists partially hydrogenated oil, avoid the product!

Red Meat

Americans eat too much red meat—we have bacon or sausage for breakfast, a hamburger or hot dog for lunch, steak for dinner, and then wake up and do it all over again.

Unfortunately, this is just not healthy! Excessive consumption of red meat has been linked to:

- Cancer (including colorectal cancer, breast cancer, prostate cancer, and pancreatic cancer)
- Diabetes
- Elevated cholesterol
- Heart disease
- Hypertension
- Chronic inflammation

In addition, red meat may contain:

- Bacteria
- Heterocyclic amines (which have been linked to cancer)
- Hormones
- PCBs (which are toxic)
- Protein prions (which have been linked to bovine spongiform encephalopathy, also known as mad cow disease)
- Viruses

Americans and other Western societies should follow the example set by people living in the Mediterranean: if you consume meat, do so less frequently (weekly or monthly, not daily), and when you do, utilize lean cuts.

High Fructose Corn Syrup

Most of us know to avoid too much table sugar, but there's an even more sinister sweetener lurking on your supermarket shelves: high fructose corn syrup. This sweetener is a favorite of the food industry since it is sweeter than ordinary table sugar, is inexpensive, and prolongs the shelf life of food. It is found in many beverages and foods, including soft drinks, sports drinks, packaged cookies, and other baked goods.

Since its introduction in 1970, the amount of high fructose corn syrup in our food has steadily increased; currently the average American consumes 73.5 pounds of this sweetener each year. Our obesity rate also jumped from 15 to 30 percent during the same period, which many nutritionists believe is not a coincidence.

The real danger posed by high fructose corn syrup, however, is the metabolic havoc it causes. In contrast to ordinary sugar, high fructose corn syrup is not utilized by the muscles as an energy source. Instead, it goes directly to the liver and leads to an increase in triglyceride production, a major risk factor for heart disease.

At a 2007 meeting of the American Chemical Society in Boston, Rutgers University researchers presented data that linked high fructose corn syrup in sodas with the development of diabetes. The research team, led by Chi-Tang Ho, PhD, found that carbonated beverages featuring the common sweetener contained high levels of highly reactive compounds known as carbonyls, according to a press release issued by the American Chemical Society. Carbonyls are chemicals that have previously been linked to a type of cellular and tissue damage implicated in triggering diabetes, and/or contributing to some of its complications.

Dairy

One of our most prevalent American myths is the health benefit of drinking three or more glasses of whole milk per day. Besides increasing cholesterol due to its saturated fat content, whole milk has been a big contributor to the obesity epidemic in America and developed nations worldwide. Note that three

8-ounce glasses of milk a day delivers 450 calories and 15 grams of saturated fat. In addition, the hormones cows are given to increase their milk production, as well as the antibiotics they're fed to prevent infection, have also been found in blood samples of milk drinkers.

Regular milk consumption may increase the risk of:

- Diabetes
- GI disturbances (due to lactose intolerance)
- Heart disease
- Multiple sclerosis
- Ovarian cancer
- Prostate cancer

If you must consume milk, enjoying fat-free or skim milk in moderation makes more sense. Likewise, choose low-fat or fat-free cheese, select low-fat or fat-free yogurt, and switch from butter and margarine to olive oil or a trans fat–free vegetable spread for your other dairy needs. Finally, for all you ice cream junkies out there, consider fat-free ice milk or a fresh fruit sorbet.

The Mediterranean Diet

In contrast, a Mediterranean diet is low in saturated and trans fats (while including necessary healthy fats), and discourages intake of refined sugar and processed foods. It's also high in the vitamins, fiber, and antioxidants required for good health, and includes many foods that have been shown to decrease inflammation, something that we know plays a pivotal role in the development and progression of heart disease, cancer, diabetes, and an increasing list of other diseases. (The typical American diet actually *promotes* inflammation.) For all these reasons, a Mediterranean diet is the basis for the diet I put all my patients on, and the diet I've been eating myself for twenty-five years.

A Mediterranean diet is characterized, generally speaking, by the foods that were available in pre–World War II Southern Europe and Northern Africa, in the countries that border the Mediterranean Sea. Think of fish and shellfish fresh from the ocean, olives and fragrant olive oil, tangy goat cheese and home-baked, whole-grain breads. Think of fresh spinach dressed with garlic, lemon, and pine nuts, or perhaps spicy hummus, the flavorful chickpea spread of the Middle East, redolent with the complex flavors of pungent garlic, bright lemon juice, and any number of tantalizing fresh herbs and spices. Think of whole-grain pasta tossed with sautéed fresh vegetables, some herbs and olive oil, or a hearty tomato sauce fresh from the garden. The beauty of the Mediterranean diet is its flexibility and diversity. Endless delicious dishes are possible, ranging from the remarkably simple to the delightfully complex.

Let's take a moment to break down the main components of a Mediterranean diet, and explain the health benefits they have to offer:

Whole Grains

Whole (non-refined) grains have been shown to decrease the risk of heart disease, diabetes, and cancer. A whole grain kernel consists of an outer layer, the bran (fiber); a middle layer (complex carbohydrates and protein); and an inner layer (vitamins, minerals, and protein). The process of refining, common outside the Mediterranean region, destroys the outer and inner layer of the grain, resulting in a stripped version that lacks the original's fiber and disease-fighting vitamins and phytochemicals.

Fresh Fruits and Vegetables

Go to any market in the Mediterranean basin and you will find a bountiful supply of fresh, native fruits and vegetables. Fruits and vegetables contain an abundance of vitamins, minerals, fiber, and complex carbohydrates that lower the risk of heart disease and cancer. They also contain phytonutrients, concentrated in fruit and vegetable skin, and antioxidants, both of which help fight disease and improve health.

Nuts

Nuts such as almonds and walnuts are rich in the monounsaturated fat and omega-3 fatty acids, which decrease inflammation and have a favorable impact on cholesterol and triglyceride levels, as well as being good sources of protein, fiber, and vitamins. Several clinical trials have demonstrated that regular nut consumption leads to lower cholesterol, lower risk of coronary heart disease, and a significant reduction in the risk of heart attack.

Beans (Legumes)

Beans are a rich source of soluble and insoluble fiber, which help curb appetite and reduce cholesterol. In addition, beans are an excellent source of protein and vitamins. Regular bean consumption has been shown to lower the risk of heart disease, cancer, and diabetes.

Fish

Oily fish provide us with a rich source of protein and, like nuts, contain high levels of omega-3 fatty acids. A warning: Several species of fish may contain high levels of mercury and other contaminants, so pregnant women and young children should exercise caution. Nevertheless, for most adults, the cardiovascular benefits of fish consumption outweigh the risks, especially if you choose fish varieties that provide the highest amount of omega-3 fatty acids and tend to contain the lowest amount of mercury. The best choices are salmon, albacore, tuna, herring, sardines, shad, trout, flounder (also known as sole), and pollock. Avoid tilefish, swordfish, shark, and king mackerel, as these fish species tend to have the highest mercury content.

Olive Oil

Olive oil, which provides the taste and flavor that is so much a part of Mediterranean dishes, is rich in monounsaturated fat, the type of fat most beneficial for heart health. The regular use of olive oil instead of butter or margarine is associated with a reduced risk of heart disease, cancer, diabetes, and inflammatory disorders like asthma and arthritis. Olive oil also has a favorable impact on cholesterol. Besides decreasing total cholesterol, it also lowers "bad" LDL cholesterol, and makes our bodies less susceptible to damage from free radicals. Olive oil also helps maintain or increase "good" HDL cholesterol, so the total cholesterol to HDL cholesterol ratio is improved.

Oleic acid, which makes up more than 70 percent of olive oil, is considerably less susceptible to oxidation because it is monounsaturated, rather than polyunsaturated like most vegetable oil fatty acids. This contributes to long shelf life and high antioxidant activity. Studies on tissue cultures and animal models of human cancer have shown that its remarkable phytochemicals work to thwart several types of cancer, through various mechanisms of action. In fact, recent research showed that oleic acid "down-regulated," or switched off, an aberrant gene involved in the promotion of many cases of breast cancer.

What's more, three of olive oil's components have been shown to have antibiotic activity against several strains of bacteria implicated in intestinal and respiratory infections, which implies, at least, that olive oil may enhance the activity of the immune system!

Red Wine

Moderate alcohol consumption has been shown to lower the risk of coronary heart disease, and red wine is believed to have several advantages over other forms of alcohol. Red wine contains polyphenols and resveratrol, two substances that help to promote heart health. Resveratrol, a powerful antioxidant, is more abundant in red wine than white wine; it lowers "bad" LDL cholesterol and raises "good" HDL cholesterol, and also decreases clotting. Remember, alcohol should be consumed in moderation: wine consumption should not exceed one to two (5-ounce) glasses per day. For those individuals who do not wish to consume wine, grape juice is an excellent alternative: grape juice—specifically purple grape juice—also lowers the risk of heart attack.

In addition to these benefits from specific foods, a Mediterranean diet generally is especially high in two other things important for good health: complex carbohydrates, and omega-3 fatty acids.

Complex Carbohydrates

Carbohydrates are a source of energy and nutrition that is essential to good health. Simple carbohydrates like candy and soda are sugars, which are quickly absorbed into our bloodstream and provide an immediate source of energy. Complex carbohydrates like whole grain bread and cereal, oatmeal, and apples are made of long strands of sugars and are broken down and metabolized more slowly, providing the body with energy over a longer period of time.

A good way to think of this is in terms of foods' glycemic index. The glycemic index is a ranking of various foods based on the speed at which those foods are able to increase blood sugar or glucose compared to white bread, which was given an arbitrary glycemic index of 100. Foods which increase blood sugar faster than white bread have a glycemic index greater than 100; foods which increase blood sugar slower than white bread are assigned a glycemic index less than 100. Carbohydrates with more fiber and less sugar have glycemic indexes less than 100, meaning that they will leave you feeling full longer. Compared to simple carbohydrates, complex carbohydrates with low glycemic indexes improve blood glucose levels and decrease your likelihood of developing diabetes and heart disease. (Fortunately, you don't need to memorize the glycemic index of food; simply by following the Mediterranean diet, you will already be consuming food with a low glycemic index.)

Omega-3 Fatty Acids

Omega-3 fat is an important component of the Mediterranean diet because it's something that the average American eater doesn't get enough of. It has been suggested that up to *90 percent* of Americans are omega-3 deficient. How can that be?

Prior to the Industrial Revolution and the migration from the farm to the city, the vast majority of our food was grown locally. Our fruits and vegetables were good sources of omega-3 fat, and since cattle were free-roaming and grass-fed, they too consumed naturally occurring omega-3, which we took in when we ate beef. Today we live in a different world. Food is shipped from farms to grocery stores, and so requires the inclusion of preservatives. Our soil has been depleted of its nutrients, and cattle are sedentary grain-fed creatures, woefully deficient in omega-3.

Why should this matter? The ratio of omega-3 to omega-6 in our body is important to health maintenance: omega-3 fat (found in nuts, olive oil, and fish) is anti-inflammatory, whereas omega-6 fat (found in corn oil and much of today's red meat) is pro-inflammatory. The omega-6/omega-3 ratio should be 1/1 to 2/1; however, due to the decrease in omega-3 intake and an increase in omega-6 intake, the omega-6/omega-3 ratio in the average American is somewhere between 10/1 to 20/1. This imbalance is associated with an increase in:

- Acne
- Allergies
- Arthritis

- Asthma
- Cancer
- Depression
- Diabetes
- Disorder of the heart rhythm
- Heart disease
- Hypertension
- Inflammatory bowel disease
- Sudden cardiac death

The Mediterranean diet alters this ratio by providing your body with ample amounts of omega-3 fat and limiting the amount of omega-6 fat you consume.

Interestingly, the components of the Mediterranean diet seem to be even more beneficial when consumed together. Their health effect is synergistic—each element builds on the others, making the diet more than just the sum of its parts.

I've adapted the traditional Mediterranean diet to our modern lifestyle, adding more foods that recent advances in nutritional science have found to be beneficial, in order to create what I call the Miami Mediterranean diet. In addition to the foods above, the Miami Mediterranean Diet also includes:

Tea

Don't let your love affair with coffee blind you from the possibility of enjoying a cup of tea. Though drinking anything containing caffeine can worsen dehydration (because they have a diuretic effect that can lead to fluid loss), one or two cups of coffee a day is fine, as long as you avoid rich, blended coffee drinks. Both coffee and tea contain antioxidants and chemicals that have been found to reduce the risk of diabetes, gallstones, and kidney stones. But it is tea that contains substances that help reduce the risk of heart disease and cancer.

Does the color of the tea matter? Both black tea and green tea come from the same source: the white-flowered *Camellia sinensis* plant, which is loaded with antioxidants and gives tea its cardiovascular benefits. Green tea may have an edge because it's made from young tea leaves, providing more antioxidant power and boosting its health benefits. But if you prefer black tea, or it's the type you have handy, don't be dissuaded from enjoying it, because it's a healthy brew as well. The same goes for white tea.

To release tea's strongest health benefits, brew it yourself, using either the leaves or a tea bag, and let it steep in the cup for three to five minutes (though different color teas may require different brewing times; check the packaging). Bear in mind that although you may enjoy herbal teas, pure tea provides more antioxidant punch.

Fruit and Vegetable Juices

Fruit juice doesn't replace the need to eat whole fruit, which has fiber and makes you feel full, but can still be a refreshing source of nutrients and disease-fighting antioxidants.

Pomegranate juice is a particularly great choice. The pomegranate's popularity is on the rise lately, thanks mostly to the growing interest in its health benefits. Like many other fruit juices, this sweet and tangy drink is loaded with a combination of antioxidants for a particularly potent effect. Research studies have found that pomegranate juice helps lower blood pressure, reduce the buildup of atherosclerotic plaque, and preserve nitric oxide, key in keeping the coronary arteries healthy. Pomegranate juice is also a great source of vitamin C and potassium, and contains less sugar than some other fruit juices. (Don't let the enthusiasm for pomegranate juice discourage you from trying the fruit itself, though; it's perfect for eating and cooking.)

Vegetable juices offer many of the same benefits as their fruity counterparts. Tomato juice and V-8, for example, are great low-calorie sources of vitamins and minerals. These juices contain a significant amount of sodium, however, which can lead to high blood pressure and fluid retention. Low-sodium tomato juice or V-8 is preferable—you can add potassium salt for taste if desired.

Beware of fruit drinks, however. Many people consume fruit drinks thinking that they are healthy, but these drinks are often nothing more than flavored sugar water, and have little to no nutritional value. Whole fruit paired with a glass of good old-fashioned water is still your best nutritional bet!

Cinnamon

Too often in America, we remove cinnamon from the cupboard only on special occasions, to flavor pumpkin pies for Thanksgiving or bake cookies during the Christmas holidays. No more! It's time to steal a secret that other countries like China and India know: that cinnamon not only flavors food, but offers health benefits as well.

Ground cinnamon is made from the bark of the cinnamon tree and it contains three types of essential oils (cinnamaldehyde, cinnamyl acetate, and cinnamyl alcohol) that provide it with health-boosting properties, as well as a wide range of other active substances. These oils have different beneficial effects: they act as an anti-coagulant, preventing blood from forming heart-attack-causing clots; they have anti-inflammatory properties; and they enhance the ability of diabetics to metabolize sugar. There's even some research indicating the smell of cinnamon can help improve brain activity.

And you don't have to down copious amounts of cinnamon to reap its benefits; research shows that less than a half-teaspoon of cinnamon a day lowers blood glucose levels and improves the cholesterol balance in people at high risk for diabetes and coronary heart disease.

Cinnamon tastes great, so it's also an inexpensive, easy way to brighten up a vast variety of recipes. Use cinnamon to spice up hot beverages, like tea or apple cider, or sprinkle it on top of sugar-free cocoa. Dust it on squash or carrots, or swirl it into yogurt and add a dash of honey for a quick dessert. Just leaf through this book and you'll find many recipes in the Miami Mediterranean diet that utilize this versatile and healthful spice. But perhaps the best tip of all is to take that container of cinnamon down from the shelf, transfer its contents to a shaker, and leave it on the kitchen table. That way, you'll keep it on hand, and use it often.

Dark Chocolate

Not everything that tastes good is bad for you. Take chocolate!

Chocolate can be enjoyed on the Miami Mediterranean diet, as long as it is dark chocolate. Chocolate is made from cocoa beans, which are one of the richest sources of beneficial antioxidants, especially flavanols. Flavanols help lower blood pressure, balance cholesterol, and maintain a favorable blood glucose level. But it is flavanols that give chocolate a bitter taste, so confectioners remove them and then add refined sugar and fat. *Viola*! The result is unhealthy milk chocolate.

Dark chocolate, on the other hand, is the darling of chocolate connoisseurs, who prefer its less sweet, more interesting taste. And thanks to its flavanols, dark chocolate also makes the grade for inclusion in the Miami Mediterranean diet, as long as it's enjoyed in moderation. Confectionary companies are catching on and touting dark chocolate's health merits. But always read the nutrition label, and choose dark chocolates that are lowest in saturated fat and sugar, have no trans fats, and contain at least 70% cocoa flavanols.

Remember, no matter how it's touted, dark chocolate still has plenty of calories, so enjoy it in moderation and, when you do indulge, don't gobble it up. Instead, savor a piece or two, perhaps with a glass of red wine, as a delightful ending to a Miami Mediterranean meal.

Unlike other diets—low-carb diets, low-fat diets, and even the American Heart Association Diet—the Miami Mediterranean diet isn't just healthier for you, it also tastes great. Though unfortunately there isn't enough space in this book for me to reprint as many suggested recipes or as extensive a meal plan as I'd like, I have included a comprehensive 7-day meal plan and nearly three dozen recipes drawn from my previous book, *The Miami Mediterranean Diet*, in Appendix C. The full book features 300 kitchen- and time-tested recipes. For more meal plans, recipes, and inspiration to get you started (and keep you committed!), I encourage you to pick up a copy.

The Mediterranean Diet and Obesity

Maintaining a healthy weight is important for many aspects of health, but weight has particular implication for cardiovascular health. Besides increasing the risk of heart attack and stroke, obesity also increases the risk of:

- Hypertension
- Type 2 diabetes
- Abnormal LDL cholesterol, HDL cholesterol, and triglycerides
- Cancer
- Gallbladder disease
- Sleep apnea syndrome
- Osteoarthritis

While many of the health implications of obesity are well known, some are less obvious. It's more difficult to diagnose early cancer in obese patients, for instance, as diagnostic imaging machines must be pushed to their limits in order to obtain images that are clear enough to interpret.

Most people are well aware that obesity is far more common

today than it was just a few decades ago. For that matter, it's more prevalent now than it was even just a few years ago, especially in this country. The United States has the highest rate of obesity in the world. It's commonly accepted that about one-third of adults are now obese, and about two-thirds of adults are overweight or obese. Researchers at Tulane University examined data from national surveys of adult health habits recently and found that the number of men and women weighing 300 pounds or more had increased from about 130,000 individuals in the study period of 1976 to 1980, to more than three *million* adults in the period from 1999 to 2004. That's a lot of excess tonnage. The trend is ominous.

Perhaps now is a good time to review some simple facts and definitions. What exactly *is* obesity? One way of quantifying obesity is through the use of the body mass index, or BMI. BMI is a number obtained by first taking an individual's weight in pounds, and dividing it by the square of his or her height in inches. Then multiply that number by 703. A five-foot-four woman who weighs 150 pounds, then, would have a BMI of around 26: $[150/(64 \times 64)] \times 703$. A BMI of $18.5 - 24.9$ is considered normal weight; $25.0 - 29.9$ is considered overweight; $30.0 - 39.9$ is obese; and anything over 40.0 is considered morbidly obese. But BMI is just a handy tool. It does not account for differences in fatty tissue versus lean muscle mass, nor does it account for the distribution patterns of excess fat.

There is evidence that certain distributions of fat—around the waist in men, for instance—are more threatening to cardiovascular health than other distribution patterns, such as weight carried in the hips, which is more common among women. Male-type, or visceral, obesity is more strongly associated with increased disease risk than the BMI alone. Waist-to-hip ratio may also be a better predictor of the risk of metabolic syndrome than BMI; anything below .8 for women and .9 for men is considered optimal. Yet another way to assess overweight and obesity is to measure percentage of body fat, but this is somewhat more difficult to calculate, and is less commonly employed.

At the most fundamental level, obesity is simply the result of more calories coming in than are being expended. Doing work—exercising for example—burns calories fairly rapidly. Sitting in front of the television or computer monitor also burns calories, but at a far slower rate. This is why recommendations to exercise and reduce calorie intake are the common denominators in virtually all (sensible) weight-loss plans.

Other factors may also play a role in the development of obesity, however. Genetics may account for at least some of the differences in how quickly different individuals store excess calories. Various environmental factors are also cited as potential contributors to the problem, particularly its increase in the population as a whole over time. Work has shifted from labor-intense to more sedentary, in keeping with our changing economy. Fast food is readily available on virtually every street corner, and we're eating it far more often. The number of families sitting down to at least one meal a day together has diminished, while the marketing of calorie-dense foods has increased. Fast-food outlets have notoriously increased their portion sizes, while prices have remained relatively steady. All of these factors may be playing at least some role in the burgeoning epidemic of obesity.

Additives such as high fructose corn syrup have been implicated by some. In fact, a recent article by researchers at the National Institute on Aging/National Institutes of Health indicates that taste receptors in the intestines may respond to some of these additives by releasing hormones that influence feelings of satiety, or "fullness," and thus influence eating behavior. We've already looked at high fructose corn syrup. Monosodium glutamate (MSG), which appears in all manner of prepared foods, ranging from Chinese takeout to canned soups and flavored tortilla chips, has in recent years been implicated in the obesity epidemic by a number of reputable scientists. While the FDA requires manufacturers to identify MSG in product labeling, other glutamate additives may hide behind innocuous-sounding names such as hydrolyzed vegetable protein or autolyzed yeast, making it still more difficult for wary consumers to avoid this potentially risky additive.

MSG is actually detected by its own unique taste-bud sensor. The taste sensation it provides is called *umami*, after an Asian word denoting the "savory" taste. Experiments on laboratory animals have shown that, when injected with MSG, animals eventually develop "significant inflammation," obesity, and type 2 diabetes. More recently, Japanese researchers found that chronic exposure to MSG in laboratory rodents resulted in the development of serious liver abnormalities similar to a human condition known as non-alcoholic fatty liver disease. "We suggest that MSG should have its safety profile re-examined and be potentially withdrawn from the food chain," the researchers concluded. Unfortunately, the vast majority of Americans are either unaware of or unconcerned by the effects of these ubiquitous additives.

The Obesity Epidemic: Not Just For Adults Anymore

Between 1980 and 2000, the number of overweight children in America—the number of children at increased risk for heart disease, high blood pressure, and diabetes, among other diseases—tripled! Overweight children have an 80 percent increased risk of growing up to be overweight adults, and it's surely no secret that overweight adults are at far higher risk of developing both diabetes and coronary heart disease. It's been estimated that one out of every six teenagers has coronary arteries that are already being affected by atheromatous plaques. And emerging evidence strongly suggests that being overweight or obese increases a person's risk of developing cancer.

In a recent article published in the influential *New England Journal of Medicine*, researchers at the University of California, San Francisco, attempted to extrapolate future coronary heart disease rates among overweight adolescents who will be 35 years old in 2020. Based on predictive models and current data about the number of overweight adolescents, the researchers concluded that heart disease rates, and deaths from heart disease, will continue to escalate if something is not done to reverse the trend toward overweight and obesity.

The Mediterranean Diet and Weight Loss

A Mediterranean diet can be a great tool for weight loss. People who live in the Mediterranean region and follow a Mediterranean diet and lifestyle are leaner than their American counterparts who consume the typical American diet.

Food consumed in a typical Mediterranean diet can lead to weight loss in a number of ways:

- The consumption of food with a high fiber content (like fruits, vegetables, beans, nuts, and whole grains) leads to high satiety—the feeling of being "full." The consumption of healthy fat (in olive oil, nuts, and fish) in the Mediterranean diet also leads to high satiety. When you feel full, you eat less.
- The consumption of omega-3 fat has also been shown to help achieve weight loss through a process known as thermogenesis (heat release following the metabolism of fat).
- The Mediterranean diet discourages simple carbohydrates and refined sugar, which have been linked with obesity.
- The Mediterranean diet also discourages trans fats, which are associated with weight gain and obesity.

Following a Mediterranean diet, while keeping portion size down and staying active (see step 2), is a great way to meet your weight loss goals while also improving your health in other ways.

What Is Wrong with the Popular Fad Diets?

Americans have always been enamored with "quick fix" diets that promise rapid, sustained weight loss. The problem with these diets is that they have no scientific basis, and there is no long-term data demonstrating their effectiveness regarding sustained weight loss or long-term health.

I consider these diets to be fad diets. Fad diets usually promise quick and easy weight loss, but the sad truth is that, although some of these diets may result in initial weight loss, the weight is quickly gained back. That initial weight loss is often not healthy weight loss, either. Starving yourself can also lead to weight loss, but it deprives you of the vitamins and nutrients you need to live, and can do permanent damage to your body.

Here's a round-up of some popular diets and their drawbacks:

LOW-FAT DIETS
The low-fat, high-carbohydrate, and mainly vegetarian diets are hard to follow, and not palatable for most Americans.

AHA (AMERICAN HEART ASSOCIATION) DIET
This low-fat diet can lead to decreased "good" HDL cholesterol, and heart disease may progress regardless. The AHA diet contains less monounsaturated fat and omega-3 fat than the Mediterranean diet, and is associated with a higher risk of heart attack and death; the Lyon Heart Study demonstrated a 73 percent reduction in cardiovascular endpoints (heart attack or death) in patients following a Mediterranean diet rather than an AHA Step 1 diet.

Low-Carbohydrate Diets

There is no long-term data demonstrating clinical benefit of following these diets, and concern about increasing the risk of heart disease and cancer make low-carbohydrate diets suspect according to many doctors. These diets are high in protein and saturated fat, and restrict carbohydrates. They do often lead to a quick, early drop in weight due to water loss, but this process of water loss can result in fluid and electrolyte changes that may lead to serious cardiac arrhythmias (heart rhythm disturbances) and kidney malfunction. The impact of these diets on cholesterol levels is unpredictable. Eating an excessive amount of saturated fat while following these diets causes some people to experience a significant rise in their "bad" LDL cholesterol—especially if they absorb cholesterol at a higher-than-average rate.

Low-carbohydrate diets that achieve an "artificial" weight loss due to water loss from glycogen breakdown and ketosis (a condition that occurs when there is a lack of carbohydrates in the diet) are usually not effective in the long run. They are, however, potentially more dangerous, which is why many doctors do not recommend them. Some of the reported side effects and complications of these diets include a potential increased risk of:

- Cancer
- Cardiac arrhythmia (disorder of the heart rhythm)
- Coronary heart disease
- Deficiency of micronutrients
- Dehydration
- Diabetes
- Elevated cholesterol
- Elevated CRP (a marker of inflammation)
- Gout
- Halitosis (bad breath)

- Impaired cognitive (memory) function
- Kidney malfunction
- Kidney stones
- Optic neuropathy

A Note on Vitamins and Supplements

Vitamins are obviously critical for optimal health. The problem with the typical American diet is that it lacks the fresh non-processed whole foods that supply us with the essential vitamins, minerals, and phytonutrients essential to good health.

The best way to get these vitamins, minerals, and nutrients is through diet; whole foods contain thousands of phytonutrients that interact with one another to achieve optimal health in a way supplements just can't replicate. Just because vitamins and other supplements should never be taken as a substitute for a healthy diet, doesn't mean they can't be helpful. A daily multivitamin that contains the recommended daily allowance for a variety of vitamins and minerals, for example, can provide a kind of "insurance policy" against nutritional gaps in your diet.

One vitamin that has recently received interest is vitamin D. A recent study published in the *Archives of Internal Medicine* found that men enrolled in the Health Professionals Follow-up Study who had a low vitamin-D level had an elevated risk for a heart attack. Vitamin D is known to affect inflammation, vascular calcification, and blood pressure. Although it has not been established that vitamin D supplementation reduces the risk of heart attack, many health care providers advise their patients to have adequate sun exposure and consume foods fortified with vitamin D. Vitamin D supplementation may also prove beneficial for cardiovascular disease prevention as well as cancer prevention, bone health, and a host of other health benefits.

A few other individual supplements you might consider taking:

Fish Oil

There is one supplement clinically proven to benefit cardiovascular health, and that is fish oil—the optimal source of omega-3 fat. Omega-3 fat (something a Mediterranean diet, unlike our American diet, is rich in) is necessary for good health, but since our body does not produce omega-3 fat on its own, we must rely on other sources. In particular, fish oil has been shown to decrease triglyceride levels.

Several large clinical trials have demonstrated the value of consuming an adequate amount of fish, either through diet or fish oil supplement. In the U.S. Physicians Health Study, it was shown individuals who consumed at least one meal of fish per week reduced their risk of sudden cardiac death by 52 percent compared to those who consumed fish only once a month. In a large Italian study, more than 10,000 men and women with preexisting heart disease were given either fish oil or a placebo. Those taking fish oil capsules had a 45 percent reduction in their risk of sudden cardiac death. A Japanese study demonstrated that the addition of fish oil to statin medication in patients with elevated cholesterol resulted in a reduced risk of heart attacks and death from heart disease compared to patients who were placed on statins alone.

One warning: High doses of fish oil may thin the blood, and so should not be taken without medical supervision.

Potassium

Potassium is an essential mineral critical for optimal heart health. When potassium levels fall in our body, we are more likely to develop high blood pressure and heart rhythm disorder. I have seen many patients over the years who were placed on blood pressure medication yet continued to suffer from elevated blood pressure. Simply increasing potassium and decreasing sodium in the diet, however, can reduce or normalize blood pressure. The same holds true for people with palpitations; often, increasing the potassium stores in the body can resolve the problem.

A word of caution: Never attempt to increase potassium on your own; elevated potassium can be just as dangerous as low potassium. People with kidney impairment need to be especially careful. Your doctor can determine your potassium level and kidney function with a blood test.

Magnesium

Magnesium, like potassium, is an essential mineral of which we often don't get enough. Magnesium lowers blood pressure and also reduces the risk of heart attack, stroke, and diabetes. It also helps to stabilize the heart rhythm. As with potassium, your doctor can check your magnesium level and discuss options and recommendations.

Coenzyme Q10

Coenzyme Q10 (CoQ10), also known as ubiquinone, is a naturally occurring antioxidant vitamin with important implications for cardiovascular health. Statin medications, used to decrease cholesterol by reducing cholesterol production in the liver, can also lead to a decrease in CoQ10. Since a reduction in CoQ10 may lead to muscle pain and discomfort, some have advocated the use of CoQ10 supplements in all patients taking statins. One study revealed that 85 percent of statin users who developed muscle pain and discomfort improved following treatment with 100 mg of CoQ10 per day.

Besides treatment for muscle pain and discomfort, preliminary evidence suggests that CoQ10 may be beneficial in the following cardiovascular conditions:

- *Hypertension*: CoQ10 causes a small reduction in blood pressure, although it's use in the treatment of hypertension remains controversial.

- *Heart failure*: CoQ10 is important for optimal mitochondrial function, an essential element in improved heart muscle contraction. Some studies have shown an improvement in heart pumping capacity following the administration of CoQ10, but other studies have not.
- *Angina pectoris (chest pain)*: Preliminary small studies suggest that CoQ10 may improve chest pain resulting from poor blood flow to the heart muscle.
- *Improved endothelial function*: CoQ10, when given to patients with coronary artery disease, resulted in an improvement in the function of endothelial cells, the cells lining the blood vessel wall.
- *Heart attack*: preliminary study suggests that CoQ10, when given within three days of a heart attack, results in clinical benefit. Further studies are needed, however, before CoQ10 is routinely recommended following a heart attack.

Although CoQ10 is generally well tolerated, it's important to discuss all treatment and prevention strategies with your treating physician.

Low-Dose Aspirin

The history of aspirin dates back thousands of years, to when the Greek physician Hippocrates used the bark and leaves of the willow tree to relieve pain and fever. The ingredient responsible for this beneficial effect was salicin—a substance that was used in 1832 to create acetyl salicylic acid, or aspirin. Soon after, aspirin was being used by physicians worldwide to treat pain, fever, and arthritis. In 1948 a California physician, Dr. Lawrence Craven, noted that 400 men to whom he prescribed aspirin did not suffer a heart attack. He advised his colleagues to use daily aspirin to reduce the risk of heart attack.

It wasn't until 1988, however, that the results of the landmark Physicians Health Study confirmed this effect. The study randomly gave over 22,000 healthy men either aspirin or a placebo, and the study was stopped early because the results were so dramatic: there was a 44 percent decrease in the risk of a first heart attack in those men given aspirin. Dr. Charles Henneckens, a renowned Harvard epidemiologist who was the lead author of this study as well as of a meta-analysis of four additional aspirin trials, noted an overall 32 percent reduction in cardiovascular events.

Aspirin's effect turned out to be less dramatic for women. The Women's Health Study, published in the *New England Journal of Medicine* in March 2005, found that low-dose aspirin (100mg on alternate days) decreased the risk of heart attack in women over the age of forty-five by 9 percent—a number that was not statistically significant. Aspirin did, however, result in a statistically significant 17 percent decrease in the risk of stroke—and a 26 percent decrease in stroke risk for women over sixty-five.

Aspirin has also been useful in treating hypertension. The HOT (Hypertension Optimal Treatment) study in 1998 demonstrated the beneficial effect of low-dose aspirin in reducing the risk of heart attack and major cardiovascular events in patients with treated and controlled hypertension.

Aspirin has proven to be especially beneficial during an active heart attack. Studies have shown a 23 percent reduction in the risk of death if aspirin is taken at the time of a heart attack. But men or women who have already had a heart attack or stroke can benefit as well. They can significantly reduce their risk of recurrent heart attack or stroke by taking aspirin on a regular basis. It should be noted, however, that there are two types of stroke: ischemic and hemorrhagic. Ischemic strokes are caused by arterial blockages or clots that shut off blood supply to an area in the brain, and aspirin is beneficial in preventing this type of stroke. The other type of stroke—hemorrhagic stroke—is caused by an arterial rupture that causes a bleed in the brain. Aspirin therapy can make this type of stroke worse. Any patient who has had a stroke should always check with their doctor before starting aspirin.

Aspirin works by thinning the blood—by preventing the aggregation or clumping of platelets, the cells that help blood form clots. Platelets contribute to clots by producing and releasing a prostaglandin called thromboxane; aspirin acts by blocking this process.

Aspirin is not for everyone. It is known that aspirin can increase the risk of bleeding, including gastrointestinal bleeding and bleeding in the brain. If you have an allergy to aspirin, asthma, gastrointestinal ulcers, inherited or acquired bleeding disorders, uncontrolled high blood pressure, reduced kidney or liver function, or a history of a hemorrhagic stroke, you should not use aspirin therapy. Nevertheless, patients who are at increased risk for heart attack and stroke, and who do not have these conditions, may indeed benefit from regular aspirin therapy.

STEP 2

Exercise Regularly

*PATIENT: Doctor, the problem with me is that obesity
runs in my family.
DOCTOR: No, the problem with you is that no one
runs in your family.*

REGULAR EXERCISE AND PHYSICAL ACTIVITY
are extremely important for heart health. Exercise is
beneficial for a number of reasons: Exercise makes
your heart stronger and more efficient, and a strong
and conditioned heart better utilizes oxygen from
your lungs than a weak or unconditioned heart. A conditioned
heart also pumps more blood with every beat, which reduces
the heart's workload and reduces its resting heart rate. Even
people who have had heart attacks can increase their chances of
survival if they include physical activity in their daily routine.
Conversely, various studies have shown that physical *inactivity*
is a risk factor for heart disease.

Professor Jeremy Morris and colleagues at the British Research Council first showed the relationship between physical
activity and heart disease in a paper published in 1953. They

studied conductors working on London's double-decker buses, who climbed around 600 stairs per workday, and compared them to bus drivers, who sat for 90 percent of the day. The conductors experienced less than half the incidence of heart attack as the sedentary drivers. Similar findings were seen in other groups: for example, postal workers who walked or bicycled on their mail routes had fewer heart attacks compared to their sedentary clerical counterparts.

Heart health isn't the only benefit of regular exercise. Regular exercise also lowers the risk of developing:

- High blood pressure
- Stroke
- Peripheral vascular disease
- Lipid disorders (such as high LDL cholesterol, low HDL cholesterol, and high triglycerides)
- Diabetes
- Metabolic syndrome
- Overweight or obesity
- Osteoporosis
- Anxiety
- Depression
- Colon cancer
- Breast cancer
- Alzheimer's disease

Many of these (including but not limited to high blood pressure and lipid disorders) have been linked to heart disease, and so in fighting them, you're gaining protection against heart disease as well.

What else can exercise do for you? Research has shown that exercise also:

- Improves bone strength
- Improves the immune system
- Increases the production of natural mood elevators called endorphins
- Improves the quality of sleep

You don't have to run a marathon or train like a prizefighter to reap the benefits of exercise; even mild exercise can be beneficial. Studies show that just ten minutes of exercise a day can boost heart health. A study done in 1996 showed that just fifteen minutes of exercise five days a week could decrease the risk of death from coronary heart disease by 46 percent. And research found that overweight or obese sedentary women who exercised 72 minutes a week increased their peak oxygen consumption (which is a measure of cardiovascular fitness) by 4.2 percent.

Walking is actually an excellent exercise (and it doesn't require expensive equipment and can be done anywhere, even in front of the TV). A study published in the 2005 issue of *Diabetes Care* demonstrated that simply walking thirty minutes a day significantly reduced the risk of dying from heart disease. Other forms of exercise, such as housework, gardening, bicycle riding, and swimming are all beneficial to your health as well.

Burning 150 calories a day through moderate exercise has been proven to reduce your risk of dying from cardiovascular disease, and for most people, walking one and a half miles a day will burn that 150 calories. (An additional benefit: 150 calories a day equals around fifteen pounds of fat a year.) A study conducted at the University of Virginia School of Medicine, reported in the *Journal of the American Heart Association*, found that men who walk more than 1.5 miles per day significantly lower their risk of heart attack compared to their more sedentary counterparts.

Though clinical studies have shown that even low levels of

activity can have short and long-term health benefits, the more exercise you do, the greater impact it has. The British Regional Heart Study involved 7,735 men between the ages of forty and fifty-nine who were studied over a period of eight years. The objective was to assess the relationship between physical exercise and the risk of heart attack. During the study, 488 men suffered at least one major heart attack. However, it was shown that the risk of heart attack decreased significantly as physical activity increased. Men who reported moderate exercise experienced less than half the risk of heart attack compared to inactive men. The study also showed that any time is a good time to start. Even men with symptomatic coronary heart disease showed a reduction in the rate of heart attack when they began exercising regularly.

The bottom line is this: daily exercise is important for maintaining optimum heart health. The good news is that regular exercise need not be vigorous or intense to be beneficial. Simply increase your daily physical activity and try to walk at least thirty minutes a day—your heart will thank you!

A Note on Aerobic Versus Isometric Exercise

Aerobic exercise is the exercise most closely tied to heart disease prevention, and refers to any form of exercise that results in a sustained increase in heart rate over a period of time. Walking, running, and swimming are all forms of aerobic exercise.

Isometric exercise refers to weight training or strength training. In isometric exercise the muscles are used to pull or push a weight, often using equipment like dumbbells, barbells, and specialized machines. It's a form of exercise that becomes critical as we get older, since we can lose up to six pounds of lean muscle mass through aging.

Isometric exercise has its own immediate benefits as well. A study by K. Cullinen and M. Caldwell published in 1998 in the

Journal of the American Dietetic Association showed that weight training decreases body fat without restricting dietary intake. Another study by A.S. Ryan and colleagues published in 1998 showed that resistance training maintains bone mineral density in post-menopausal women.

Most exercise experts recommend a combination of both aerobic and isometric exercise for maintaining good health.

Manage Your Stress

Stress is not having to sink a three-foot putt for $100,000—it's having to sink a three-foot putt for a dollar when you only have 50 cents in your pocket.

—LEE TREVINO, Professional Golfer

NOT LONG AGO I was reading an article in a prestigious cardiology journal that discussed risk factors for heart disease. Cholesterol, blood pressure, smoking, and other factors were discussed in great detail. There was just one problem with this article: stress was never mentioned!

I consider stress to be the "forgotten" risk factor. It's easy to measure blood pressure and cholesterol. But how do you measure stress? In addition, what is stressful for one person may not be stressful for another. Because of all this, the negative impact of chronic stress on long-term health is often underappreciated by health care providers. Stress reduction strategies are rarely discussed with patients at the time of their office visit. But stress's impact on heart disease can be huge. The INTER-HEART study, recently reported in the journal *Lancet*, examined stress at home, at work, and due to major life events in more than 27,000 people. The study found that stress raised heart attack risk more than 2.5 times—an increase similar to that of smoking and diabetes!

Stress is a natural part of living. In fact, the stress response used to be essential for our survival. When a caveman was attacked by a saber-tooth tiger, he needed a sudden surge of adrenaline in order to fight or flee. The problem for modern man (and woman) is when stress becomes constant. Chronic stress increases stress hormones, such as cortisol and adrenaline, which in turn increase blood pressure, cholesterol, and blood sugar, cause the heartbeat to become rapid, and increase the "stickiness" of our platelets, which increases the likelihood of blood clots. The net result of chronic stress for modern man is an increased risk of heart attack and stroke.

Financial Stress

One of the most frequent stressors I encounter in heart attack patients is their financial situation. A Consumer Federation of American analysis of Federal Reserve data revealed that the average American household is approximately $10,000 to $12,000 in debt and uses up to nine credit cards. In the last two decades, credit card debt has nearly tripled. With this in mind, one can easily see how the burden of financial stress has become an added health risk factor affecting millions of Americans. In fact, a study from Ohio State University concluded that people with high credit card debt relative to their overall income are more likely to suffer from health problems. Even subjects who followed a healthy diet and who exercised regularly still experienced increased health issues.

There are many approaches to achieving financial freedom and avoiding monetary stress, and many books you can pick up to help. But here are a few basics: Live within your means.

Don't use more than one credit card. Maintain a monetary reserve for unexpected emergencies. And start saving for retirement and your children's college educations now.

Don't let financial stress eat at you! A heart attack could be the result.

Are You a Hot Reactor?

People who are impatient and become upset with minor everyday stress are "hot reactors," a term coined by the late cardiologist Dr. Robert Elliot. "Hot reactors" are individuals who have extreme cardiovascular responses to stressful situations—people who react so strongly to stress that their bodies produce especially large amounts of stress chemicals. This results in a profound cardiovascular response, such as a rapid rise in blood pressure and heart rate. This response can occur over and over during the day even due to common stressful situations.

Hot reactors are at greater risk for developing stress-related cardiovascular diseases such as heart attack and sudden cardiac death. Treatment for these individuals may require not just lifestyle changes, but medication and psychological counseling.

Handling Stress

How you handle daily stress is the key to keeping stress hormones under control. There are lots of things you can do to manage your stress. I've included a handful below, but my list is far from comprehensive. The important thing is that you find something that relaxes you, and make sure you make the time to do it!

Just Breathe

Easier said than done, right? But it's easier to do than you'd think. There is a natural flow in your body between the stress response, and something called the relaxation response. This give and take occurs unconsciously and is influenced by several factors: your breathing, your level of activity, and your state of arousal.

Dr. Herbert Benson, a professor at Harvard Medical School and the founder of the Mind-Body Institute in Boston, developed a technique to harness the relaxation response. It's a simple approach that takes ten to twenty minutes and involves only a few steps:

1. Find a comfortable and quiet place.
2. Close your eyes and try to relax your muscles.
3. Breathe deeply in and out in a natural and rhythmic way, while silently chanting a word (such as "peace") with each breath.

You can encourage the relaxation response in other ways as well. Another approach to relaxation is slow, deep breathing.

Imagine you are in the office, sitting at your desk and quietly working, when you are suddenly faced with an unexpected, difficult task. Your breathing becomes more rapid and your heart rate and blood pressure rise as increased stress hormones are released into your bloodstream. By taking back control of your breathing, you can influence the rest of the stress response as well. Inhale slowly, hold your breath for a few seconds, and then slowly exhale. Repeat this process several times until your breathing slows and you feel more relaxed and in control. As you repeat this process, your heart rate and blood pressure will also normalize. This simple approach can be done by anyone, anywhere, to help reduce a stress response.

For some people, choosing a soothing word to repeat mentally as they slowly inhale and exhale helps them to achieve a sense of serenity and return to a less stressful state.

Slow, rhythmic breathing is a common denominator in many spiritual practices. Let's look at a few of the most popular.

Meditation

In meditation, you focus on a word, a sound, a symbol, or your own breathing in order to calm your mind and body. One variation is mental visualization or guided imagery, in which you focus on a pleasant, comforting image or a scene where you feel at peace. Typically, this kind of meditation works best in a quiet and comfortable setting. Both traditional meditation and mental visualization have shown to be beneficial methods for stress management and stress reduction.

Self-Hypnosis

Self-hypnosis is another way to induce relaxation. First, change into comfortable clothing, and then find a quiet place with a comfortable chair and play soft calming music. Start with slow deep breathing, starting your inhalation deep in your abdomen and imagining each breath is on a journey through your body, slowly spreading from your toes to your fingertips before finally being exhaled. Repeat this breathing exercise over and over as you begin to relax. Then let your thoughts take you to a place that you find calming, or one that makes you feel good. Imagine, for example, you are in a beautiful forest with birds singing and beautiful flowers that fill the air with sweet fragrance. As you walk among the trees and flowers, you go deeper and deeper into the serene calmness of the forest, leaving your current surroundings and stress far behind. The result is a feeling similar to daydreaming or deep concentration. When you end your journey and return to full consciousness, you should feel more relaxed, calmer, and further removed from your daily stresses.

Yoga

The ancient art of yoga has been practiced for more than 5,000 years. While yoga emerged in Eastern countries, it has recently become popular in the West; the benefits of yoga have even been adopted by many companies in America and Europe that recognize that relaxed workers are healthier and more creative.

The basic principles of yoga include:

1. Deep breathing
2. Physical movement and stretching
3. Meditation
4. Mental visualization or guided imagery

Yoga's aim is to bring together the mind and body. The use of physical movement, different poses, and stretches, along with breathing techniques, allows both the mind and body to relax.

There are various styles of yoga to choose from. Some are more aerobic and work up a sweat, while others are slower and more spiritual in nature. Research done at Boston University School of Medicine and McLean Hospital, reported in the May 2007 issue of the *Journal of Alternative and Complementary Medicine*, suggested that the practice of yoga may elevate levels of gamma-amino butyric (GABA), the brain's primary inhibitory neurotransmitter. Those elevated GABA levels may help to reduce anxiety and depression.

Exercise

Exercise has actually proved to be the best method for relieving tension, a true remedy for stress. A recent review of exercise and its relationship to anxiety, depression, self-esteem, mood, and emotion was done by the National Consensus on Physical Activity and Mental Health. Their conclusion was that exercise appeared to reduce anxiety and stress both in single sessions and when engaged in regularly.

A randomized controlled trial conducted by Duke University Medical Center concluded that exercise training and stress management helped to reduce cardiovascular risk. Another study, a randomized controlled trial by Blumenthal et al reported in the

Journal of the American Medical Association in 2005, concluded that patients with coronary heart disease who exercised and had stress management training reduced stress and improved markers associated with cardiovascular risk more than conventional medical care alone.

Several mechanisms have been proposed for how exercise reduces stress. First, regular exercise lowers adrenaline levels, leading to a lower heart rate, lower blood pressure, and a sense of calm. Second, exercise stimulates the release of endorphins, the "feel good" brain hormone that leads to a natural high. Third, regular exercise like walking or swimming allows people to forget their daily stress by focusing on repetitive movement.

Napping

Believe it or not, napping too has been shown to reduce stress. For some reason our culture frowns on the idea of midday naps for anyone other than small children. But many adults also experience a natural decrease in alertness after eight hours of working, particularly if they don't get enough nighttime sleep.

It is natural to feel drowsy in the afternoon, and research has shown that a brief nap can result in greater alertness, reduced levels of stress, and improved cognitive function. A NASA study showed that a short nap boosted airline pilots' performances by 33 percent.

In fact, a midday catnap can recharge your batteries better than drinking a strong cup of coffee: studies have shown that people who power nap get better results on memory tests than those who drink caffeine. And a fifteen to thirty minute nap in the afternoon seems to provide more benefits than even longer nighttime sleep—though most experts feel that sleeping beyond thirty minutes puts you into a deeper stage of sleep and makes it more difficult for you to fall asleep at night.

Some corporations have introduced power nap rooms for their employees. In New York City one can even find "sleep pod centers" where weary people can come off the street and settle into a hooded, pod-shaped chair for a few minutes or more of peaceful rest.

One recent study showed that people who take a regular midday nap cut their risk of dying from a heart attack by 37 percent. But even if you only have five minutes to spare, just close your eyes and relax. Even a brief rest reduces stress and provides added energy to get you through the day.

Relationships

Love and happiness are essential to good health. Studies have shown that a strong supportive social network of both family and friends not only helps us survive the tough times in life but also helps us fully enjoy the happy ones. In addition, such supportive relationships have been associated with lower levels of stress and longer lives. Unfortunately, the reverse is also true— a stressful relationship has an inverse impact on longevity.

The lack of meaningful personal relationships, or "social isolationism," is another strong stress producer. Numerous studies have demonstrated the link between social isolation and increased mortality rate, especially following a heart attack.

One way to increase your interpersonal (or in this case, interspecies) relationships is to get a pet. Owning a dog or a cat may be just what the doctor ordered to help you reduce your level of stress. A study done in 1990 showed that elderly people who had dogs or cats as pets made fewer visits to their doctors. Another study conducted at the State University of New York at Buffalo found that people on medication for hypertension reduced their blood pressure when they got a pet. Still another study demonstrated that owning a dog is associated with prolonged life after heart attack.

Pets are also great motivation to exercise, adding even more stress reduction effect. Taking your dog for a walk is not only good for the dog, it's good for you too!

Hobbies

Hobbies provide an outlet—a way to "blow off steam"—as well as take your mind off of what's going on in the rest of your life. They've been shown to lower stress levels, improve mood, and reduce depression. A study conducted in Turkey found that doctors who did not have outside interests or hobbies had the highest rates of depression. Another research study showed that men who did not have hobbies had a higher incidence of illness and more frequent absenteeism from the workplace.

Music

Music is an effective stress reducer in both healthy people and those with health issues. Students who listened to classical music while engaged in a stressful task were shown to have reduced anxiety, lower heart rates, and lower blood pressure. A study in the *Journal of Applied Social Psychology* found that men and women who drove their car in congested traffic (a classic stressful situation) while listening to music had less stress than those who did not listen to music.

Prayer

Prayer may also be an effective way to reduce stress. An article published in the journal *Progress in Cardiovascular Nursing* in 2002 stated, "Complementary therapies and healing practices have been found to reduce stress, anxiety, and lifestyle patterns known to contribute to cardiovascular disease. Promising therapies include . . . prayer."

Another article, from the March 2006 issue of the *Journal of Atherosclerotic Reports*, commented on the recent INTERHEART Study, which reported that psychosocial stress accounted for about 30 percent of the attributable risk for acute myocardial infarction. It stated that psychosocial stress is a highly modifiable risk factor that can be reduced by, among other things, prayer.

Laughter

Laughter may very well be the best medicine. There is strong evidence that laughter can actually improve health and help fight disease. "Laughter, along with an active sense of humor, may help protect against a heart attack," say researchers at the University of Maryland Medical Center in Baltimore, who recently conducted a study on the health benefits of laughter. The study indicated that people with heart disease laughed less often in response to everyday situations and displayed more anger and hostility than people of the same age who did not have heart disease. I have noticed over the years myself that my patients who had a good sense of humor and enjoyed a good laugh had fewer heart attacks and lived longer.

One study demonstrated that neuroendocrine and stress-related hormones decrease during periods of laughter. According to psychologist Steve Sultanoff, PhD, president of the American Association for Therapeutic Humor, "With deep, heartfelt laughter, it appears that serum cortisol, which is a hormone that is secreted when we're under stress, is decreased." Another study that linked the therapeutic benefits of laughter to health was conducted by researchers at Loma Linda University in California. The study has linked laughter to lower blood pressure, a reduction in stress hormones, an increase in muscle flexion, and a boost in the function of the immune system.

The mere expectation of laughter makes you feel good as well. An interesting study split a group of sixteen people into two groups. One group was told that they would be watching a funny movie and the other group (the control group) was not. Blood was drawn from all subjects just before the video was started. The subjects who were told they were going to see a funny movie had 27 percent more beta-endorphins (the feel-good hormone) in their blood sample than those subjects in the control group. The elevated levels of beta-endorphins remained elevated in the group during the video and continued to be elevated for twelve to twenty-four hours afterward. It was concluded that these results, combined with other research on how laughter improves mood, appear to show positive implications for wellness, disease prevention, and stress reduction.

Laughter even has a beneficial impact directly on blood vessels. Research done at the University of Maryland Medical Center in Baltimore suggested that laughing was almost as beneficial as exercise in boosting the health of blood vessels. The investigators showed that laughter relaxes arteries and increases blood flow, suggesting that laughter could help keep the artery lining healthy and help to reduce the risk of cardiovascular disease. Some scientists have hypothesized that laughter releases chemicals that are protective to the artery lining, preventing cholesterol from entering the wall to form the plaques that cause heart attack. Michael Miller, MD, director of the University of Maryland's center for preventative cardiology, has said, "Because we know of many more factors that contribute to heart disease than factors that protect against it, the ability to laugh—either naturally or as a learned behavior—may have important implications in certain societies such as the United States, where heart disease remains the number one killer. . . . Thirty minutes of exercise three times a week and fifteen minutes of hearty laughter each day should be part of a healthy lifestyle."

Laughter also has a positive effect on diabetes. Keiko Hayashi, PhD, R.N., of the University of Tsukuba in Ibaraki, Japan, conducted a study involving nineteen people with type 2 diabetes. The results showed that laughter lowers blood sugar. Blood was collected from the patients before and two hours after a meal. On the first night the patients were shown a boring forty-minute lecture after dinner; on the second night they were shown a forty-minute comedy show. Blood sugar was significantly lower after the comedy show.

Research conducted at Graz University in Austria suggests that laughter is beneficial for stroke patients as well. Thirty

stroke patients were split into two groups. One group partici-
pated in regular "laughter yoga" sessions for six weeks while
the other group did movement exercises only. Blood pressure
levels remained roughly the same in the movement group but
dropped significantly in the laughter group. Mood improved in
both groups, but it was more noticeable in the laughter group.
Participants in the laughter group also said they felt more awake
and less stressed. Psychologist Ilona Papousek, who headed the
research, said, "This is the first study that shows that laughter
has an effect on blood pressure."

Finally, a recent study presented at the American Society
of Hypertension 2008 Annual Meeting in New Orleans found
that "laughter yoga," a blend of laughter, deep breathing, and
stretching, significantly lowered both systolic and diastolic
blood pressure. Cortisol, a hormone released during times of
stress, was also lowered. There are currently more than 6,000
laughter clubs in sixty countries.

A Positive Outlook

The power of positive thinking—the belief that the glass is
half-full rather than half-empty—has important health benefits. There are studies that show that one thing people who live
long and healthy lives have in common is their positive atti-
tude. One interesting study conducted in Minnesota on nuns
with Alzheimer's disease showed that nuns with a positive outlook lived ten years longer than those who expressed negative
emotions.

When it comes to stress, the glass is definitely half-full—just keep
a positive outlook, and find your own ways to reduce stress.

STEP 4

Take Command
of Your Blood Pressure

YOUR BLOOD PRESSURE is the measure of the force of your blood against the artery walls, and it is described using two numbers: systolic and diastolic. Systolic pressure is the pressure exerted as your heart beats; diastolic pressure is the pressure exerted as your heart relaxes between beats. A normal blood pressure reading used to be less than 140/90 mmHg, with 120/80 mmHg as the ideal. But recent changes in the guidelines set normal as less than 120/80 mmHg.

It is normal for your blood pressure to fluctuate during the day due to physical activity or stressful stimuli; it should return to normal as your body adjusts to whatever situation you're in. If it does not, if your blood pressure is chronically elevated to greater than 140/90 mmHg, then the condition is called hypertension. Hypertension is unfortunately common, affecting more than 50 million Americans.

We used to think that only diastolic pressure was an important predictor of cardiovascular events, but it is now understood that both numbers matter. Elevated systolic pressure is a key indicator of stroke risk, especially in the elderly. Left uncontrolled, it can also result in kidney disease, vascular disease, and increased risk of heart attack.

The most common cause of hypertension is aging. Blood vessels lose their elasticity as we age, and that reduction in the ability to expand and contract can lead to a rise in systolic pressure and a decrease in diastolic pressure. A young, healthy artery reacts just like a balloon would in response to increased pressure—it expands. Older arteries aren't always flexible enough to do so, which means blood ends up pressing against the artery wall with greater force.

Another common cause of hypertension is heredity predisposition. Someone with a strong family history of hypertension is at higher risk of developing hypertension later in life than someone with no family history.

Hypertension that is caused by certain treatable conditions is called secondary hypertension. Nutritional causes are surprisingly common. One question I always ask patients is if they eat licorice. Licorice contains glycyrrhizin, a substance that may cause sodium retention and lead to hypertension. Excessive salt, alcohol, and caffeine can also increase blood pressure. Decreasing or eliminating these from the diet can do a lot to reverse hypertension.

Other secondary causes of hypertension may be reversible through surgery. These include constriction of the aorta, a tumor on the adrenal gland, or a blocked renal artery. People who also snore may have obstructive sleep apnea, a cause of hypertension that has several treatment options.

In other words, even if you're leading a healthy lifestyle, you could still develop hypertension. This is why a complete evaluation by your personal physician is necessary. Diagnosing and eliminating any secondary causes can significantly reduce or even eliminate hypertension altogether.

If you have no secondary causes, however, the best way to

treat hypertension is with lifestyle changes, even if you also need medications. I recommend a four-part program for all my patients with high blood pressure, consisting of:

1. Nutrition
2. Exercise
3. Stress management
4. Smoking cessation

Nutrition

From years of clinical studies, we know a lot about the impact of various foods on blood pressure. Fruits and vegetables, for example, are particularly rich in phytonutrients, which we've learned help lower blood pressure. In fact, all the foods essential to the Mediterranean diet discussed in step 1—fruits and vegetables, whole grains, olive oil, cold-water fish, red wine, nuts, and beans—have been shown to help lower blood pressure. There are also specific foods you should stay away from because of their negative effects on blood pressure: saturated fat, trans fat, and sodium. In addition, excessive consumption of caffeine and alcohol can lead to a rise in blood pressure.

My first recommendation here is to follow a Mediterranean diet. But you can also add individual foods to your diet that contribute to reducing blood pressure. Green tea contains catechins, antioxidants that inhibit the action of an enzyme responsible for raising blood pressure. Pomegranate juice has recently gained attention for its ability to lower blood pressure as well as inhibit atheromatous plaque formation. Even chocolate can be beneficial if you eat the right kind and limit the amount. Moderate consumption of a small amount of dark chocolate, rich in flavanols, contributes to healthy blood vessels, which ultimately leads to reduced blood pressure.

Increasing your intake of potassium, magnesium, and calcium may also have a beneficial effect. Supplements are one way to this, but you can also just choose foods rich in these minerals. Foods that contain a lot of potassium include tomatoes, bananas, blueberries, and oranges. Foods that contain a lot of magnesium include nuts, seeds, beans, fish, whole grains, and green vegetables. And dairy products are a particularly rich source of calcium.

Exercise

Exercise lowers blood pressure in a few ways. One way is by supporting weight loss, particularly the reduction of abdominal fat. Fat in this area is associated with elevated levels of a protein called angiotensinogen, which can lead to hypertension. Exercise also strengthens the heart and makes the cardiovascular system more efficient by relaxing and dilating blood vessels. And if you exercise instead of raiding the refrigerator as an outlet for stress, you can both eliminate emotional eating and help yourself maintain a healthy weight. As mentioned in step 2, simply walking thirty to forty-five minutes each day can lead to significant benefits.

Stress Management

Stress releases catecholamines, chemicals that prepare the body for physical activity and can raise blood pressure. See step 3 for suggestions for reducing stress.

Smoking Cessation

Cigarette smoking causes arteries to constrict and contributes to blood pressure elevation. Smoking's negative health impact, and some tips for quitting, is covered more in-depth in step 7 in the discussion on toxins.

If you currently smoke, stop. No amount of smoking is safe, and it is counterproductive to an otherwise healthy lifestyle.

Medical Therapy

If lifestyle changes are not sufficient to control your blood pressure on their own, medications can be a useful tool. The more common medications used to lower blood pressure include:

- Thiazide diuretics
- Angiotensin converting enzyme (ACE) inhibitors
- Angiotensin receptor blockers (ARBs)
- Calcium channel blockers
- Beta blockers

See the chart and details in chapter 5 for more information.

In addition, new blood pressure lowering medications, such as direct renin inhibitors, are now available. Single pills or capsules which contain various combinations of medications from different classes have also been developed.

The decision to use a specific medication should be individualized. If a patient has hypertension and asthma, for instance, a beta blocker would not be a wise choice, as blocking the effects of adrenaline can make asthma worse. A beta blocker may be a smart choice, however, for a patient with hypertension and a rapid heartbeat, since it can slow the heart rate and decrease palpitations.

It is also important to remember that many prescription and non-prescription medications can cause or exacerbate hypertension. For instance, common over-the-counter medications taken for pain and inflammation such as nonsteroidal anti-inflammatory drugs or NSAIDs like Advil® and Aleve® may raise blood pressure. Always read the label and warnings on medications and supplements you take and discuss possible side effects with your health care provider.

STEP 5

Control Your Cholesterol

We've never had a heart attack in Framingham in 35 years in anyone who had a cholesterol level under 150.... Three quarters of the people who live on the face of the Earth never have a heart attack. They live in Asia, Africa and South America, and their cholesterols are all around 150.

—Dr. William Castelli, Medical Director,
Framingham Cardiovascular Institute

CHOLESTEROL CONTROL is really the first line of defense against heart disease, since the development of atherosclerosis begins with "bad" LDL cholesterol. Remember how atheromatous plaques are created? LDL cholesterol in the bloodstream penetrates the artery lining and is trapped in the artery wall. There, it starts the process that can ultimately lead to heart attack and stroke. But the lower your cholesterol is, the less likely LDL cholesterol is to leave the bloodstream in the first place. Lower your cholesterol, and lower your risk of heart disease.

But how low is low enough? The average total cholesterol in American men and women is 208 mg/dl. Compare that to what we've learned is the optimal cholesterol level—less than 150 mg/dl! Where did we get 150? From the Framingham Heart Trial—the multi-decade study of lifestyle and dietary habits we looked at back in chapter 2. Dr. William Castelli, the trial's former director, used the term "150 club" to refer to the level of cholesterol below which he did not find a heart attack in any of the trial's subjects.

The average "bad" LDL cholesterol in American men and women is 130 mg/dl; it should be less than 70 mg/dl. When we are born, our average LDL cholesterol is only 35 mg/dl. It is our toxic diet and lifestyle that causes this number to more than triple by the time we reach adulthood. The cholesterol level of hunter-gatherer tribes, for instance, is much lower: their LDL was only 50 to 70 mg/dl, and they averaged a total cholesterol of 110 to 130 mg/dl. Notably, they didn't develop atherosclerosis or suffer heart attacks. (See step 9 for more information on advanced cholesterol testing and optimal cholesterol levels!)

Lowering Your Cholesterol

What we need to do is clear: reduce our total cholesterol to under 150 mg/dl, and our LDL cholesterol to less than 70 mg/dl. Luckily, how to do it is just as clear. Cholesterol in our body comes from two sources: what we eat and what we produce. We can lower our blood cholesterol levels by decreasing our consumption of foods containing cholesterol, saturated fat, and trans fat. Today we can also lower cholesterol levels by taking medications such as statins that decrease the production of cholesterol.

The top foods that have been shown to have a favorable impact on cholesterol, by lowering the "bad" LDL cholesterol or by raising the "good" HDL cholesterol, include:

- Fruits and vegetables
- Olive oil
- Oatmeal
- Nuts (especially almonds and walnuts)
- Beans
- Cold water fish
- Red wine
- Cinnamon
- Whole grains
- Soy protein
- Plant sterol and stanol spreads

The fiber contained in fruits and vegetables lowers cholesterol; in addition, plant sterols in fruits and vegetables interfere with cholesterol's intestinal absorption. The fiber in nuts, and the plant sterol and stanol in spreads, work the same way. The omega-3 in fish lowers triglycerides, red wine raises "good" HDL cholesterol, and cinnamon (and olive oil) lowers "bad" LDL cholesterol. You may recognize this list of foods from step 1; they're also the main components of a Mediterranean diet.

In addition, exercise has been shown to raise "good" HDL cholesterol, lower triglycerides, and make the "bad" LDL cholesterol particles larger. Larger LDL particles, you'll recall from chapter 2, are less likely than smaller particles to squeeze through the artery lining, get trapped in the wall, become oxidized, and form plaques.

Another option is cholesterol-lowering medication. Despite a heart-healthy diet and exercise program, some men and women still have elevated "bad" LDL cholesterol, reduced "good" HDL cholesterol, or elevated triglyceride levels. These individuals usually have an inherited genetic basis for their abnormal cholesterol and can benefit from medical therapy in addition to diet and exercise.

How Low Should We Go?

The current cholesterol treatment guidelines are based on risk factors for cardiovascular disease (see appendix B). I would nevertheless argue that everyone should strive to achieve a total cholesterol less than 150, a "bad" LDL cholesterol less than 70, a "good" HDL cholesterol greater than 50, and a triglyceride level less than 100 through diet and exercise.

If these numbers cannot be achieved with lifestyle intervention, then the decision to begin medications should be discussed between the patient and his or her personal treating physician, based on risk factors for developing cardiovascular disease. If your doctor decides to put you on cholesterol-lowering medication, there are a couple of popular options:

- Statins
- Resins
- Niacin
- Cholesterol absorption inhibitor

See the chart and details in chapter 5, and appendix B, for more information.

All that said, while cholesterol medication has helped millions of people, it's only a useful secondary tool, not something that "makes up" for unhealthy behavior! Medications are *not* a substitute for lifestyle changes.

STEP 6

Reduce Free Radicals and Oxidative Stress

THE FORMATION OF ATHEROMATOUS PLAQUES, the dangerous cholesterol-laden deposits that can lead to heart attack and stroke, begins when LDL cholesterol gets into the artery wall. But what happens next is just as key to plaque formation as cholesterol itself. Inside the artery wall, LDL cholesterol comes into contact with free radicals, those electron-stealing byproducts of cellular respiration we talked about in chapter 2, and becomes oxidized, kicking off a potentially dangerous immune response as the body registers the oxidized cholesterol as a foreign invader.

Ready for some bad news? First, cholesterol isn't the only thing free radicals steal electrons from. Left unchecked, free radicals cause damage on the cellular level in every part of the body. They've been shown to play a part in everything from this book's subject, heart disease, to premature aging, cancer, and many other diseases. When they steal electrons from cholesterol, it leads to heart disease; when they steal electrons from DNA, it leads to cancer.

Second, oxygen free radicals aren't the only free radicals floating around your body, looking for electrons to steal. We know from Part I that oxygen free radicals are produced as a normal part of cellular respiration—the process of turning food into energy—and are used by the immune system to fight off foreign invaders (you can read about this process in more detail, as well, in appendix B). But any molecule can become a free radical. All the term "free radical" means is that the atom or molecule is missing an electron and looking for a new one to replace it. So when an oxygen free radical steals an electron and becomes stable—no longer a free radical—whatever molecule it stole from usually becomes a free radical in its place. The new free radical then steals an electron from something else, and so on, creating a dangerous chain reaction that causes disease.

Third, there are certain things—toxins—that, when they enter the body, cause free radical production to go into overdrive. Exactly why this happens, scientists don't yet know. What we do know is that introducing toxins into the body is like adding lighter fluid to a fire—it causes a free radical explosion.

Known toxins include air pollutants (like carbon monoxide from car exhaust), ultraviolet rays, pesticides, and radiation (from X-rays and tests like the CAT scan as well as things like your television and computer screens). Things like cigarette smoke, excess alcohol, the preservatives and additives in processed foods, and trans fats are also toxins, in that they ratchet up free radical production. It's impossible to get away from toxins altogether, though we do have some control over the amount of exposure we receive. And we are exposed to many, many more toxins today than our ancestors were even fifty years ago.

Here's the good news: We know how to fight free radicals. We can abstain from smoking (including passive smoking from inhaling the smoke of cigarette smokers), and avoid exposure to air pollution and unnecessary ionizing radiation (see chapter 6). Most importantly, we can avoid the highly processed and calorie-dense toxic American diet that leads to free radical production. We have a way to make free radicals stable and stop the chain reaction of free radical creation. That way is antioxidants.

Antioxidants

Antioxidants—which include vitamins and nutrients like vitamins C and E, and beta-carotene—work by supplying free radicals with the extra electron they would otherwise steal from cholesterol or DNA or other cells of the body. Antioxidants, however, can lose an electron to a free radical without becoming free radicals themselves.

One way to think of it is as if there were a war going on inside your body, all the time. On one side are the free radicals, which are attacking your cells; on the other side are the antioxidants, which are trying to "neutralize" the free radicals before they can cause any damage. The more antioxidant soldiers you have, the better off you are.

Unfortunately, we don't manufacture many antioxidants on our own. Rather, we get most of them from the foods we eat— largely fruits and vegetables, but also whole grains, beans, and other plant products. Despite our best efforts, we haven't been able to duplicate the benefits of a healthy diet simply by taking a few pills. Different antioxidants work at different "levels" of the cells in our body: some of them protect cell nuclei, for instance, while others protect cell membranes. And we need thousands of different antioxidants in order for our whole body to remain healthy. The best way to ensure this happens is to eat a wide range of fruits and vegetables, in a variety of colors, as the different food colors bring a wide variety of free radical-fighting antioxidants to the table.

For example:

- Oranges provide vitamin C
- Tomatoes provide lycopene

- Carrots provide beta-carotene
- Blueberries provide anthocyanins
- Spinach provides lutein and zeaxanthin
- Purple grapes provide resveratrol

One intriguing experiment, reported recently in the *Journal of the Federation of American Societies for Experimental Biology*, demonstrated the benefits of antioxidants, specifically resveratrol (found in red wine as well as in purple grapes). One group of subjects was given a simple meal of turkey cutlets. A second group was given 200 mL (about 6.8 fluid ounces) of red wine with the turkey cutlets. And a third group was given turkey cutlets that had been pre-soaked in red wine before cooking, in addition to the 6.8 ounces of wine.

Afterward, the investigators measured post-meal oxidative stress by assessing blood levels of malondialdehyde, a toxic compound involved in oxidative stress. Even though turkey is *not* high in saturated fat, which is ordinarily associated with heart disease, eating a simple turkey cutlet was sufficient to raise blood levels of malondialdehyde alarmingly. However, researchers found that the group who also drank the red wine reduced their post-meal oxidative stress dramatically in comparison— and the oxidative stress in the group whose meat had also been pre-soaked was reduced to *zero*. This experiment demonstrated a simple concept: by consuming ordinary foods, such as turkey, our bodies inevitably generate free radicals . . . *unless* there are plenty of antioxidants ingested in the same meal.

If you're looking for a way other than red wine to increase your antioxidant intake, green tea could be a great choice. Green tea is a rich source of antioxidants called catechins. The best known and most prevalent of these, epigallocatechin gallate (EGCG), is so efficient as an antioxidant that it actually protects the body from the damaging effects of ultraviolet radiation. This effect has been proven, not only when green tea extract is applied directly to the skin, but also when it is consumed orally. Laboratory studies and clinical trials have indicated that EGCG and/or green tea extract may offer protection against various forms of cancer, including prostate, breast, and oral cancer, and that it may alleviate symptoms of rheumatoid arthritis and protect against the development of Alzheimer's disease, among other potential benefits. These findings are not surprising, given that many of these conditions are believed to be related to oxidative stress.

Even better than green tea, however, may be pomegranates. Pomegranates have received considerable attention due to their powerful antioxidant capacity; they show promise in improving atherosclerosis-related conditions such as erectile dysfunction in men, and are effective at preventing cell damage from oxidation. A recent objective analysis conducted by researchers at UCLA examined the relative antioxidant capacity of various widely available antioxidant drinks, including green tea, white tea, red wine, and grape, cranberry, orange, and pomegranate juices. Results confirmed manufacturers' claims that pomegranate juice offers the highest antioxidant potency of any of the beverages tested.

But wait—there's a fruit that may offer even more antioxidant prowess than the pomegranate: the Muscadine grape. The Muscadine grape is native to the Southeastern United States and is harvested mostly from August through mid to late October. They are well adapted to a warm climate and have a natural resistance to disease. The Muscadine grape differs from other grapes in several ways. The most notable difference is size: the Muscadine grape is noticeably larger than other grapes, measuring from 1-inch to more than 1-1/2 inches in diameter. Its skin is also thicker than that of other grapes—and as we know, it's the skin of most fruits and vegetables that contains most of the disease-fighting phytonutrients. Perhaps the best feature of the Muscadine grape is its antioxidant punch—it has more than five times more resveratrol than other grapes, and has more antioxidant power than cranberries, blueberries, or even, yes, pomegranates, according to the USDA.

Cocoa and the curry spice turmeric are other great examples of natural antioxidants. Cocoa has been shown to directly benefit endothelial function, and to lower blood pressure, possibly through antioxidant activities. Turmeric, the canary-yellow spice that is a fundamental component of Asian curries, is the source of highly beneficial antioxidants called curcuminoids. The most common of these, curcumin, has been avidly studied in recent years due to its apparent ability to suppress cancer at various stages, among numerous other beneficial activities, including anti-inflammatory activity. Current human clinical trials are investigating the role of this ancient spice/herbal medicine in treating everything from atherosclerosis, to colon cancer and multiple myeloma, to psoriasis, high cholesterol, and Alzheimer's disease.

In the war for your health, your body is the battleground. By avoiding toxins and eating high antioxidant foods, you can help stop free radicals before they cause the oxidative stress that leads to heart disease, cancer, and other disease.

A Note on Smoking

There are 2.4 million deaths each year in the United States, and nearly 400,000 of those deaths are related to cigarette smoking. That's roughly one in every six. Clearly, smoking is a major public health hazard.

Cigarette smoking increases free radicals. Tobacco smoke contains more than 4,000 chemical compounds, many of which are known toxins. The tar in tobacco consists of multiple chemicals that have been shown to contribute to cancer. And as we just saw, the more toxins you introduce to your body, the more free radicals are produced—which means more oxidized cholesterol, and the development of more atheromatous plaques.

Smokers have a 70 percent greater risk of dying from coronary artery disease than non-smokers. But smoking doesn't contribute only to heart disease. Studies have also shown that cigarette smoking contributes to a higher risk of developing lung cancer, chronic obstructive pulmonary disease, stroke, and peripheral vascular disease. The nicotine in cigarettes causes an increase in blood pressure, forcing the heart to work harder. Carbon monoxide in cigarette smoke takes the place of oxygen in the blood, so the heart has to beat faster to deliver enough oxygen to the rest of your body. In fact, cigarette smoking is so notorious for its role in causing disease that the Surgeon General called it "the leading preventable cause of disease and death in the United States."

Quitting Smoking

The nicotine in cigarettes causes a chemical addiction, and is one reason smokers become dependent on them. But smoking can also be a behavioral habit. Many smokers become used to lighting up a cigarette every time they have a cup of coffee or an alcoholic drink, making it harder for them to stop. In addition, many people who smoke claim that smoking relaxes them and relieves stress.

Five Basic Steps to Help You Quit

- *Get ready*. This means removing all cigarettes from your home, car, office, and anywhere else you spend time. Don't let others smoke in your home. And get rid of ashtrays, lighters, and matches; they'll just remind you of what you're trying to stay away from.
- *Find support and encouragement*. Tell friends, family, and co-workers that you are quitting and ask them to support your efforts. Tell your personal physician and other health care providers, and join a support group.
- *Learn how to fight the urge*. Get involved in a new sport

or hobby, like walking, playing tennis, or painting. Find something to do *instead* of lighting up that cigarette. Staying busy will give you less time to think about your cravings.

- *Get medication and use it correctly.* There are lots of products out there to help you stop smoking and lessen the urge. Take advantage of them!
- *Keep at it.* If you relapse, don't despair, just try again. Many people try several times before they succeed.

STEP 7

Avoid Chronic Inflammation

Atherosclerosis is not a bland lipid storage disease—
it is a chronic inflammatory disease.

—DR. PETER LIBBY, Harvard Medical School

S O FAR WE'VE LOOKED AT TWO WAYS we can affect the metabolic processes that lead to heart disease:
lowering cholesterol, and preventing cholesterol oxidation by fighting free radicals. Here's a third: avoiding
chronic inflammation.

After cholesterol trapped in the artery wall is oxidized by
free radicals, the immune system sends inflammatory cells to
attack. This inflammatory response is what causes a plaque to
form, as white blood cells surround and engulf the oxidized
cholesterol, which is perceived as a foreign invader.

The stronger your body's inflammatory response—the more
white blood cells you have inside a plaque, releasing the proteinases that eat away at the plaque's fibrous cap and the tissue
factor that causes blood to clot—the more likely your plaques
are to rupture and cause dangerous blood clots that lead to
heart attacks. But that's not the only way inflammation's been

linked to heart disease. Chronic inflammation may inhibit the release of nitric oxide, the chemical responsible for the dilation of blood vessels, leading to narrowed arteries, decreased blood flow, and increased blood pressure.

Essentially, what we've learned is that inflammation is involved in all stages of coronary artery disease, from the initiation of the plaque in the artery wall, to the plaque's progression and rupture, to the clot that blocks blood flow to the heart muscle, resulting in heart attack.

There are many reasons chronic inflammation may occur. One is simply the presence of oxidized cholesterol in the artery wall. But there are several other causes of inflammation that should be addressed:

Diet

The first one is diet. As it turns out, there are many aspects of the typical American diet that are pro-inflammatory—that actually *promote* inflammation. Red meat, omega-6 fat, trans fat, and high fructose corn syrup particularly contribute to increased inflammation in the body. In contrast, the foods included in a Mediterranean diet tend to be anti-inflammatory—they *reduce* inflammation. Fish, omega-3 fat, olive oil, and walnuts have all been shown to fight inflammation.

Disease

There are also a number of diseases that result in a state of chronic inflammation, which then leads to increased risk of heart attack or stroke. Examples include arthritis, chronic bronchitis, and chronic prostatitis (inflammation of the prostate gland), and periodontal disease (an inflammation affecting the tissues that surround and support the teeth). Treating these conditions, whether with lifestyle changes or medication (in many cases, antibiotics and anti-inflammatory medications are required), is a necessary first step toward keeping systemic inflammation low.

Obesity

Most people feel that obesity is strictly a cosmetic problem. Unfortunately, this isn't the case. One of the hallmarks of obesity is chronic low-grade inflammation—elevated levels of inflammatory markers, such as interleukin-6, and tumor necrosis factor-alpha. It turns out that these inflammatory markers are actually produced, in part, by fat cells—especially abdominal fat cells.

A Sedentary Lifestyle

A sedentary lifestyle is also directly correlated with a low-grade inflammatory state. Conversely, as exercise increases, inflammation tends to decrease. I have seen numerous overweight or obese patients who had elevated inflammation levels lower these levels thanks to beginning an exercise program. Whether the lowering of inflammation levels is directly related to exercise or whether it's related to weight loss associated with exercise, however, is not fully known.

Whatever the cause, chronic inflammation is dangerous. However, with an anti-inflammatory diet, regular visits to your doctor to catch and treat any inflammatory diseases, and regular exercise, you can do a lot to keep inflammation from increasing your risk of heart attack and stroke.

Anti-Inflammatory Medications

Certain medications that reduce chronic inflammation have been shown to reduce the risk of heart attack. Aspirin is an example: besides blocking platelets and lowering the risk of blood clots, it also reduces inflammation by targeting and deactivating enzymes responsible for promoting inflammation, specifically COX-1 and COX-2. These enzymes assist in converting a chemical derived from food, in particular omega-6 fatty acids, into various pro-inflammatory compounds.

Other drugs that work similarly—and are referred to as non-steroidal anti-inflammatory drugs, or NSAIDs—such as ibuprofen and naproxen, also inhibit the activity of either COX-1, COX-2, or both. Unfortunately these drugs don't decrease the risk of heart attack—they may even increase it.

It's interesting to note that the omega-3 fatty acids docosa-hexanoic acid (DHA) and eicosapentaenoic acid (EPA), commonly obtained through the diet by eating fatty fish, act like natural anti-inflammatory compounds in the body. In fact, fascinating research published in the past few years has revealed that these essential nutrients are converted by the body to new-found families of anti-inflammatory compounds called *protectins* and *resolvins*, which put the brakes on inflammation before it spirals out of control. As if the information in step 1 didn't give you enough reason to increase your omega-3 intake!

There is ongoing research to develop new medications that target and inhibit specific inflammatory proteins involved in atherosclerosis. For example, there is a third enzyme, 5-lipooxygenase or 5-LOX, which few anti-inflammatory drugs target, and which therefore presents an important opportunity for future medical intervention.

STEP 8

Prevent Metabolic Syndrome and Diabetes

W HY SHOULD WE STRIVE to prevent diabetes and metabolic syndrome? The answer is simple: These conditions lead to premature heart attack, stroke, and vascular disease. In fact, diabetes is considered a coronary heart disease risk equivalent—which means that diabetics have the same risk for a future heart attack as men and women who have had prior heart attacks!

Metabolic Syndrome

One in every four Americans has metabolic syndrome, a condition of metabolic derangement characterized by three or more of the following:

1. Abdominal obesity (waist size > 40 inches for men and > 35 inches for women)
2. High fasting glucose (> 100 mg/dl)
3. High blood pressure (> 130/85 mmHg)
4. Elevated triglycerides (> 150 mg/dl)

5. Low "good" HDL cholesterol (< 40 for men and < 50 for women)

We've seen how most of these factors place you at increased risk for cardiovascular disease individually (and we'll look at high glucose later in this step, when we talk about diabetes), and why they should be avoided. But metabolic syndrome is more dangerous than just the sum of its parts: it is associated with an even greater risk of cardiovascular risk than these individual disorders combined, and is considered a distinct entity by many doctors and scientists.

Metabolic syndrome is a relatively modern phenomenon, and many scientists believe that its abrupt rise in most industrialized countries is related to obesity and lack of exercise. In addition to its association with cardiovascular disease (some scientists even refer to it as *cardio*metabolic syndrome), it is particularly associated with increased risk of insulin resistance... and type 2 diabetes.

Type 2 Diabetes

Diabetes is an abnormal condition defined as a fasting blood sugar in excess of 125 mg/dl (100 mg/dl or less is normal). Symptoms may include increased thirst, increased hunger, weight gain or loss, frequent urination, fatigue or exhaustion, delayed healing of cuts or sores, and blurred vision. Some people may not exhibit these symptoms at all, or they may have only minor or insignificant symptoms. Only a physical exam and blood test can diagnose diabetes for sure.

There are three main types of diabetes:

- *Type 1 diabetes*, which usually appears in childhood or adolescence and is characterized by a defect in the cells in the pancreas that manufacture insulin. This type of diabetes is generally believed to be related to auto-immune factors or possibly a virus.

- *Type 2 diabetes*, which usually appears in adults and is caused by insulin resistance (in which cells become resistant or less responsive to insulin). This type of diabetes has been increasing worldwide and is believed to be caused by poor nutrition, lack of exercise, and weight gain.
- *Gestational diabetes*, which appears during pregnancy and usually does not continue afterward.

Why is insulin so important? Insulin is a hormone, produced by specialized cells in the pancreas, that plays a crucial part in our cells' ability to process sugar. In effect, insulin works like a key, "unlocking" cells and allowing glucose to go inside, where it's utilized as an energy source or stored as glycogen. Without insulin, glucose remains in the bloodstream, and cells aren't able to produce the energy they need to survive. This is why type 1 diabetics are treated with insulin injections: the injections provide their bodies with the insulin their pancreas does not.

In the case of insulin resistance and type 2 diabetes, it's as if someone has gummed up the locks, and so the key no longer works as well. Initially the body may compensate by producing more and more insulin. But in time, the cells producing the insulin may "burn out." Insulin production diminishes, and that causes blood sugar levels to rise.

This excess of blood sugar is known as *hyperglycemia*. When cells are not able to get the glucose they need, they are forced to use other substrates for energy, such as fatty acids (derived from the breakdown of triglycerides). Elevated blood glucose levels can lead to advanced glycation end products, or AGEs, in the blood vessel wall that stimulate the inflammatory cells to release proteinases. As we have learned, proteinases can weaken the fibrous cap of an atherosclerotic plaque, leading to plaque rupture and heart attack. In addition, this excess blood glucose wreaks havoc on small capillaries and nerves. Left unchecked, hyperglycemia can lead to serious tissue damage. In the retina the damage may eventually lead to blindness. In the kidneys it may eventually lead to kidney failure, and the need for regular dialysis to prevent the buildup of life-threatening toxins in the bloodstream. The extremities are another common site of degeneration. The nerve and small-vessel damage there may lead to pain and discomfort, and eventually severe tissue damage, especially in the feet. Amputations are not uncommon in such cases.

Unfortunately, the prevalence of diabetes is on the rise. In fact, according to a recent report by a Harvard-based researcher, the incidence of type 2 diabetes among Americans more than doubled between 1980 and 2004.

Obesity, Diabetes, and Metabolic Syndrome

In step 7 we talked briefly about obesity's tie to inflammation: how fat cells actually secrete inflammatory markers, called adipokines, indicating a direct link between the two conditions. Let's return to this concept, to see how obesity is also connected to metabolic syndrome and diabetes.

The discovery of adipokines, and their production by fat cells, has led to a revolution in our conceptual understanding of fat. Fat, it seems, is not merely an inactive blob—a static place to store excess lipids in the form of triglycerides. Instead, fat, especially abdominal fat, appears to be an influential endocrine organ that may have less in common with the gallbladder, which serves a purely repository function, and far more in common with structures like the adrenal glands, which excrete powerful hormones that exert control over numerous functions in our bodies.

By extension, this means that as fat's mass increases, its influence over the rest of the body increases as well. Organs and tissues affected by the adipokines that fat secretes include, among others, blood vessels and the immune system. In fact, some experts now view abdominal fat as the biggest endocrine organ in the body.

By the time fat has increased to the point of obesity, it begins to cause metabolic dysfunction, including insulin resistance and high blood pressure. And recent research indicates that the influence of fat cell-produced adipokines may extend beyond metabolic effects to include everything from immunity to cancer and bone formation.

Your fat may be trying to control you in other ways, as well. Adipose fat tissue's primary "goal" appears to be adding to its own mass. Part of adipokines' function is to mediate the satiety—the feeling of fullness that ordinarily results from having consumed a sufficient amount of food. Excess adipokines in your body cause this natural weight control mechanism to malfunction.

The one adipokine that *decreases* with obesity, adiponectin, ordinarily acts to reduce inflammation and promote healthy function of the artery lining. Decreased secretion of adiponectin and the accompanying dysfunction of the artery lining may eventually lead to hypertension and increased risk for heart disease, as LDL cholesterol is allowed to more easily enter the artery wall.

Some of the inflammatory compounds fat cells secrete have also been directly or implicitly linked to the development of insulin resistance. In 2001, scientists announced the discovery of a new protein, produced primarily by fat cells, that appears to impair glucose tolerance and insulin activity. Appropriately dubbed "resistin," this fat-generated protein is believed by some researchers to play a role in the development of insulin resistance and diabetes, although this remains controversial.

Suffice it to say that obesity, metabolic syndrome, and diabetes are intricately linked.

Prevention

The good news is, metabolic syndrome and type 2 diabetes can be prevented! And you'll be unsurprised by this point to learn that our best weapons in fighting and defeating these conditions are not scalpels or medications, but lifestyle changes—although medications are useful if changes in diet and activity alone are not successful. (Patients with type 1 diabetes can also benefit from following a healthy lifestyle, although they will always need insulin therapy, since they suffer from reduced insulin production rather than insulin resistance.)

One of the key studies to highlight the importance of diet and exercise for the prevention of type 2 diabetes was the Diabetes Prevention Program (DPP). This major clinical trial separated more than 3,000 overweight patients with high fasting glucose (fasting glucose between 100 and 125) into two groups. The first group, the lifestyle intervention group, received instructions regarding diet, exercise, and behavior modification. The second group took metformin, a diabetes medication designed to lower blood sugar.

The results of this trial were astounding: 58 percent of the patients assigned to the lifestyle intervention group reduced their risk of developing diabetes. An even more impressive 71 percent of those participants over age sixty reduced their diabetes risk. The metformin group also benefited, but not nearly as much as the lifestyle intervention group: they reduced their risk of developing diabetes by only 31 percent.

A healthy diet is the first step toward preventing or reversing both metabolic syndrome and diabetes. Something else that shouldn't surprise you by now: A recent study from Spain, published in the *British Medical Journal* in May 2008, found that people who follow a Mediterranean-style diet are less likely to develop new-onset diabetes. Over 13,000 healthy men and women were enrolled in this study, which lasted 4.4 years. Participants who adhered most closely to a Mediterranean diet were 83 percent less likely to develop diabetes compared to those who did not follow a Mediterranean diet.

Numerous oral medications have been developed to treat diabetes and lower blood sugar, and additional advances have been made in its treatment and management. Some act by increasing insulin secretion, while others improve insulin sensitivity. As well, research surrounding the transplant of insulin-producing cells in the pancreas has progressed rapidly over the past decade. But the optimal approach for the treatment and prevention of type 2 diabetes still remains lifestyle changes—diet and exercise that lead to weight control and an improvement in insulin sensitivity, culminating in a patient who no longer suffers from either metabolic syndrome or type 2 diabetes.

Have an Annual Physical Exam with Comprehensive Lab

MOST PEOPLE GO TO THEIR DOCTOR only when they get sick. They wait until they have a medical catastrophe like a heart attack or stroke, believing that their doctor will meet them in the emergency room and "fix" the problem. But by that point, it's often too late.

The best way to avoid expensive, life-changing medical disasters is to uncover issues *before* they irrevocably affect your health. Rather than wait for disaster to strike, visit your doctor on an annual basis, when you're healthy. Your doctor will start by getting your medical history and performing a physical exam. Then he or she should also do a comprehensive blood test to uncover any hidden risks.

I've listed details specific to heart disease screening below.

The Medical History

A proper medical history includes the following:

- Present illness (a description of how you feel and any significant recent symptoms, such as chest pain or shortness of breath)
- Past medical history
- Family history (a family history of a premature heart attack or stroke is a significant risk factor for heart disease)
- Social history (marital status, occupation, etc.)
- Medications
- Allergies
- Review of systems (symptoms reported by the patient related to the heart, lung, gastrointestinal tract, etc.)

The Physical Exam

A physical exam can quickly uncover abnormalities. Some of the important signs of cardiovascular diseases that your doctor should look for include:

EYES
- Is there evidence of retinopathy (disease of the retinal blood vessels), suggesting hypertension or atherosclerosis?

BLOOD PRESSURE
- Is it elevated, indicating hypertension (high blood pressure), or is it too low, indicating hypotension (low blood pressure)?
- Is there a difference in blood pressure between the right and left arms or between the arms and legs?

JUGULAR VEINS
- Are the neck veins distended, suggesting heart failure?

CAROTID ARTERIES

- Is there a carotid bruit (a sound heard with the stethoscope), suggesting a carotid artery blockage?

PULSE

- Is the pulse regular?
- Are the pulses in the ankles and feet decreased or absent, suggesting a blockage in the arteries in the legs?

LUNGS

- Are the lungs clear or is there fluid, suggesting congestive heart failure?

HEART

- Is there a heart murmur, suggesting a heart valve problem?

ABDOMEN

- Is there a pulsating mass, suggesting an abdominal aortic aneurysm?

LEGS

- Is there swelling, suggesting fluid retention or congestive heart failure?
- Is there pain or swelling on only one side, suggesting a blood clot in the veins?
- Is there loss of sensation, suggesting nerve damage from diabetes?

The Comprehensive Blood Test

Blood tests are a useful way of detecting problems that may not have manifested yet as physical symptoms, and of determining the correct cause of what physical symptoms are already present. We'll talk about just a few that are particularly useful in determining heart disease risk.

The Advanced Lipid Test

The most important blood test for determining metabolic cardiovascular risk factors is the advanced lipid test. There are advanced lipid tests currently done by a few different companies: the VAP (Vertical Auto Profile) test (Atherotech), the NMR Lipoprofile (Liposcience), and the Berkley gradient gel electrophoresis test. I usually recommend the VAP test, because it has generally been the least expensive, but it doesn't matter which one you use; they all provide the extra data you and your doctor need to put together an effective prevention plan.

Advanced lipid testing is performed just like a traditional cholesterol panel. A technician or nurse draws blood and submits it to a laboratory. But the test provides significantly more information than routine cholesterol tests, expanding on the traditional test's results as well as looking at additional factors. As a result, advanced lipid testing generally detects 90 percent of those at risk for heart disease—more than twice that of routine cholesterol panels!

I have performed advanced lipid testing on many patients who have already had heart attacks or strokes, or who have undergone heart procedures such as bypass surgery or stent placement. The results have often led me to think that if advanced lipid testing had been performed earlier, the patient's heart attack or stroke may have been prevented, or surgery may not have been necessary.

The expanded information from advanced lipid testing includes:

TOTAL CHOLESTEROL
The total amount of cholesterol in your blood, in all cholesterol-carrying particles. (Optimal Goal: <150 mg/dl)

LDL CHOLESTEROL
The total amount of cholesterol found in LDL particles. LDL, or low-density lipoprotein, is a main carrier of cholesterol

through the bloodstream. Elevated levels are considered a primary cause of heart disease. LDL is the primary cholesterol target in heart disease risk management. (Optimal Goal: <70 mg/dl)

HDL CHOLESTEROL

The total amount of cholesterol found in HDL particles. HDL, or high-density lipoprotein, is also a carrier of cholesterol through the bloodstream. HDL is considered protective to the cardiovascular system, due to its ability to remove cholesterol from the artery wall. Low levels are associated with increased risk for coronary heart disease. (Optimal Goal: >50 mg/dl)

TRIGLYCERIDES

The total amount of triglycerides found in triglyceride-carrying particles. Triglycerides are energy-rich molecules needed for normal functions throughout the body, but elevated levels are associated with diabetes and cardiovascular disease. (Optimal Goal: <100 mg/dl)

VLDL

VLDL, or very low-density lipoprotein, is a carrier for triglycerides. Elevated levels are a risk factor for heart disease.

NON-HDL CHOLESTEROL

The sum of the cholesterol found in all cholesterol-carrying particles except HDL. Elevated levels are a better predictor of heart disease risk than LDL alone.

LP(A)

Lipoprotein(a) is a type of small dense LDL, and is an inherited risk factor for heart disease. It is more dangerous than other types of cholesterol-carrying particles, and does not respond to traditional LDL-lowering drugs.

IDL

IDL, or intermediate-density lipoprotein, is an inherited risk factor for heart disease. It is often elevated in patients with a family history of diabetes.

LDL SIZE

The size of your LDL particles, reported in terms of "pattern" (Pattern A particles are large and buoyant, where as Pattern B particles are small and dense). Smaller LDL particles are associated with increased risk for heart disease because they enter the artery wall more frequently and are more likely to be oxidized.

HDL SIZE

The size of your HDL particles, reported in terms of "subclass" where HDL2 is larger than HDL3. Smaller HDL particles are associated with increased risk for heart disease because they are less capable of removing cholesterol from artery walls.

VLDL SIZE

Smaller VLDL particles are associated with increased risk for coronary heart disease.

The National Cholesterol Education Program recommends people begin regular cholesterol testing at age twenty. Unlike CAT scans, there is no risk in being tested, just an additional cost. Even if you are healthy, if you can afford it, you should consider having the test done. Learning about your cardiovascular disease risk early in life will allow you to take aggressive steps now—including diet and exercise—to maintain a healthy heart for life.

Baby boomers, who have taken more hands-on responsibility for their health than any previous generation, can be even

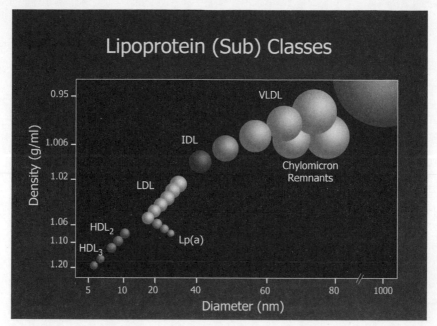

Figure 9: Lipoproteins come in a range of sizes and densities.

more strongly motivated to adopt wellness strategies when they better understand the specific risks facing them. It is one thing to tell patients their cholesterol is high and they need to reduce it. It is something else to tell them they can decrease their risk of heart attacks and emergency room visits by implementing specific strategies to adjust specific cholesterol particles. The more definitively a health threat can be identified, the greater patients' compliance with treatment is likely to be.

The Particle Number Test

There is another cholesterol factor that is important and that is particle number. Your doctor can measure the total number of bad cholesterol-carrying particles and the total number of good cholesterol-carrying particles in your blood. The total number of bad particles (LDL, IDL, VLDL, LP(a)) is more predictive of coronary heart disease risk than simply measuring LDL choles-

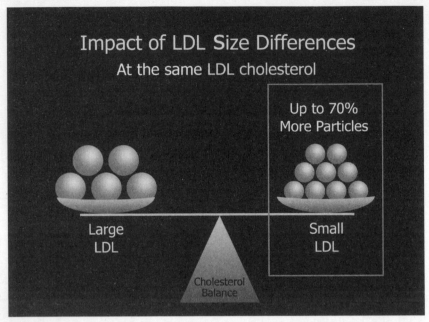

Figure 10: Two people with the same level of cholesterol may have different levels of risk due to the number of particles carrying that cholesterol through their bloodstream.

terol alone. Likewise, the higher your number of "good" HDL particles, the lower your risk for coronary heart disease.

While your "bad" LDL cholesterol level may be normal, you could still have elevated particle numbers—which means that your LDL cholesterol is distributed across a lot of very small, dense particles. A great way to visualize this is to think of the amount of LDL cholesterol in your body as the amount of space in a trashcan. You can fill the trashcan up with basketballs (large particles) or you can fill it up with ping pong balls (small particles); either way, it occupies the same amount of space. Unfortunately, small, dense LDL particles are the most dangerous kind—they are more likely to squeeze through the lining of the artery and more likely to become oxidized once they're there.

You can check your "bad" particle number by testing the

blood for apolipoprotein B (or apoB) level, or by using nuclear magnetic resonance (NMR), a specialized test that measures particle number. Likewise, you can measure the number of "good" particles using a blood test that measures the apolipoprotein A1 (or apoA1) level. Either way, knowing your particle number can save your life.

Other Tests

Inflammation can also be evaluated with blood tests. High levels of inflammatory proteins indicate increased risk for cardiovascular disease, and vascular-specific inflammatory risk markers, including high sensitivity CRP and LpPlA2, should particularly be checked. (Inflammation and its relation to heart disease are covered in detail in step 7.)

In addition to the advanced lipid test, particle number test, and tests for inflammatory markers, your doctor should also test your homocysteine level. The homocysteine level, if elevated, increases the risk of cardiovascular disease and blood clotting. While B vitamins (specifically folic acid, B6, and B12) have been shown to lower homocysteine levels, taking them in pill form has *not* been shown to lower the risk of cardiovascular events such as heart attack or stroke. A healthy diet that contains rich sources of the necessary B vitamins (such as fruits, green leafy vegetables, nuts, whole grains, and fortified cereals) is a better approach.

In addition, new emerging risk markers, such as the omega-3 index, have been developed and may be worth testing for. The omega-3 index measures the amounts of the omega-3 fatty acids present in red blood cells. Because these essential fatty acids are so crucial to cardiovascular health, it's been proposed that a low omega-3 index may indicate an increased cardiovascular disease risk.

But when I do blood tests for my own patients, in addition to doing an advanced lipid profile, I always test for the number of good and bad particles, high-sensitivity CRP, and LP(a). These three tests are the most important for uncovering hidden risk for heart attack, stroke, and vascular disease, thereby allowing physicians to target treatment programs that will best lower their patients' risk of death and disability from cardiovascular disease.

STEP 10

Avoid Unnecessary Diagnostic Tests and Procedures

ILL WAS A HEALTHY and happy fifty-four-year-old who enjoyed playing tennis and was active in his real estate business. His wife saw an ad in the newspaper that read "spend a little cash and save your life—get a coronary calcium scan." Since this ad was placed in the newspaper by the local hospital, for Bill's fifty-fifth birthday his wife paid $350 for a coronary calcium scan that would detect any "hidden" problems in Bill's heart. Sure enough, Bill was told that he had calcification in one of his coronary arteries.

Bill had always been healthy, but now he was frightened. His family physician sent him to a cardiologist, who immediately recommended a nuclear stress test. Following the stress test, Bill was informed that he had a mild decrease in blood flow at the distribution of his left anterior descending artery, and told that a heart catheterization was needed to exclude a coronary blockage. Now Bill was petrified.

During the heart catheterization, a 75 percent blockage was discovered in Bill's mid-left anterior descending artery, and a coated stent was used to open the blockage. The cardiologist went to the waiting room and exclaimed, "Bill is a lucky man. We got there just in time and fixed the problem." Bill's wife hugged the cardiologist and thanked him for saving Bill's life. A follow-up stress test performed two months later again suggested a mild decrease in blood flow to Bill's heart, and Bill was advised to get another heart catheterization. He refused to have another invasive procedure done and demanded a second opinion.

When I saw Bill six months later, he was anxious and depressed. He had quit playing tennis and he was having a hard time sleeping at night. Bill was now convinced that he would drop dead from a heart attack at any moment. "Prior to all these tests," he explained, "I felt well, had no chest pain, and enjoyed life. But since I went through all those procedures, I no longer enjoy life, I'm depressed, and I'm certainly not any healthier. In addition, I have to take blood thinning pills for the rest of my life. The medical bills are piling up; I already owe more than $50,000!"

Did Bill really need that coronary calcium scan? Definitely not! He was happy and healthy and now he is a cardiac cripple. The diagnostic procedure simply served to send Bill down a slippery slope that led to more and more unnecessary interventions.

Diagnostic Tests

To treat a patient, a doctor first needs to find out what is wrong. One of the chief tools for doing so is the diagnostic test. After listening to the patient describe his or her symptoms and performing a physical exam, the doctor decides what test or tests would be most useful in obtaining a diagnosis.

The best diagnostic tests are those that are inexpensive, safe, quick, easy to perform, and provide information that can usefully affect the management of the patient. Three diagnostic tests cardiologists often order that give the "biggest bang for the buck," for example, are blood tests, the electrocardiogram (or EKG), and the echocardiogram. Since cardiovascular disease is a metabolic disorder, proper blood testing can uncover dangerous metabolic issues likely to lead to heart attack or stroke. An EKG gives the doctor a quick look at the heart and can be used to evaluate chest pain, heart rhythm disorder, and a variety of other heart-related disturbances. The echocardiogram uses sound waves to create a two- or three-dimensional picture of the heart while it's beating in a way that is safe, painless, and relatively inexpensive, and can be performed in a matter of minutes. Best of all, there is no radiation exposure and no IV required, and it can be used to diagnose numerous heart disorders.

Compare these to a few of the less useful yet over-utilized diagnostic tests. In chapter 6 we talked about a few common cardiovascular tests that are not only unnecessary, but actually cause damage to the body. We'll start with a quick review of those, and then take a look at two others.

64-Slice CAT Scan

The 64-slice CAT scan is the newest diagnostic test available. It is promoted as a quick and easy way to see inside the coronary arteries and screen for blockage, and properly used, it is a wonderful new technology. In the case of a patient in the emergency room with chest pain, where time is essential, it can quickly distinguish a blocked artery from a blood clot in the pulmonary artery from a dissection of the aorta.

However, the value of this diagnostic tool falls apart when it is used to screen symptomless patients for coronary artery disease. The 64-slice CAT scan exposes the patient to a high dose of radiation, increasing the risk of cancer. And there is no evidence that obtaining a 64-slice CAT scan lowers the risk of heart attack or death in men and women who have no symptoms.

Nuclear Stress Test

The treadmill exercise test has been used for decades to evaluate patients' response to exercise. A patient is connected to an EKG monitor and blood pressure cuff, and walks on the treadmill while the EKG and blood pressure are monitored. This kind of stress test can uncover many cardiovascular disorders, including:

- Inadequate blood flow to the heart muscle (usually) due to coronary blockage
- Heart rhythm disorder
- High blood pressure response to exercise
- Low level of aerobic fitness

The nuclear stress test was developed to allow cardiologists to see the blood flow to the heart as well as monitor the EKG response to exercise, thereby increasing the accuracy of the test. Unfortunately the patient must receive a dose of radioactive material through an IV for that to happen. The patient becomes "radioactive," which increases the patient's risk of cancer.

The second pitfall of the nuclear stress test is that any abnormal finding usually leads to other tests and procedures, usually tests and procedures that studies have not shown to reduce the risk of either heart attack or death.

Coronary Calcium Scan

Coronary calcium scans have not been recommended by the American Heart Association or the American College of Cardiology for mass screening of men and women—yet they continue to be promoted by doctors, hospitals, and outpatient clinics, and by advertisements in the newspaper as well as on radio and TV.

Coronary calcium scans are X-ray studies, done with special CAT scanners, that detect the amount of calcium in the artery wall. The proponents of coronary calcium scans claim that the more calcium you have in your arteries, the greater your risk of heart attack, making the test key to determining treatment. Detractors state that coronary calcium scans do not provide any useful information that cannot be obtained through patient history, physical exam, and blood tests. Furthermore, there are other tests that provide additional information regarding the risk of a heart attack at a fraction of a coronary calcium scan's cost. (An example is the ankle-brachial index, a simple test that compares the blood pressure in the upper and lower extremities.)

The two most disconcerting aspects of coronary calcium scans, however, involve the scans' potential risk. First, the scans expose the patient to unnecessary radiation. As explained in chapter 6 in the discussion on CAT scans, radiation exposure increases the risk of cancer. While this scan does expose the patient to less radiation than other cardiac CAT scans, there is no dose of radiation that can be considered safe.

The second risk with coronary calcium scans is the potential for unnecessary heart catheterization and surgery. Often patients are told that they need additional tests because of the presence of calcium in the artery wall, leading eventually to unnecessary heart surgery. Conversely, the patient with a normal scan can be lulled into a state of complacency: why should they stop smoking and start exercising if their scan is normal?

Cardiac Catheterization

Cardiac catheterization can be a useful and essential diagnostic procedure in the unstable patient to evaluate the coronary arteries and heart muscle function. Unfortunately this test is also an over-utilized procedure in stable patients. In cardiac catheterization, a long thin tube, or catheter, is inserted, usually via the femoral artery in the groin. The catheter is then advanced under X-ray guidance to the heart, where it is positioned into the left main coronary artery and right coronary artery. Pictures of the coronary arteries can then be taken by injecting an iodi-nated contrast agent. The catheter is then advanced to the left ventricle and iodine is again injected through the catheter in order to take images of the left ventricular motion. Sounds sim-ple enough. In fact, millions of these procedures are performed every year. The question is, is cardiac catheterization really that simple—and is it really necessary?

I don't consider cardiac catheterization to be either simple or risk-free. It is an invasive procedure, more akin to surgery than image scanning, that can lead to deadly complications, and it should not be ordered at the drop of a hat.

Some of the potential complications of cardiac catheteriza-tion include:

- Rupture or dissection of the coronary artery requiring emergency open heart surgery
- Cardiac arrest (especially during coronary or left ventric-ular angiography)
- Iodine-induced allergic reactions
- Iodine-induced kidney failure
- Femoral artery aneurysm and bleeding
- Infection and sepsis
- Radiation exposure
- Air embolism and stroke

The most common complication of cardiac catheterization, however, is the inappropriate treatment that follows the proce-dure. Patients are often informed prior to the procedure that if a coronary blockage is found, a stent will be inserted to prop the vessel open. As we saw in chapter 4, this approach is flawed—with few exceptions, there is no evidence that opening a partially or completely blocked coronary artery in stable patients will pre-vent a future heart attack or prolong life. In fact, the insertion of a stent may actually increase the risk of heart attack and death.

Cardiac catheterization also serves as an excuse to move stable patients to the operating room for coronary artery bypass surgery. Like stent placement, this approach is flawed, since the majority of patients will do better with lifestyle changes and medical therapy than surgery.

Dr. Thomas Graboys of Harvard Medical School saw 168 patients who were told that they needed cardiac catheterization and who came to him for a second opinion. He concluded, in the study published in the *Journal of the American Medical Association* in 1992, that 162 of the 168 patients did not need cardiac catheterization. While cardiac catheterization is an essential diagnostic tool in unstable patients or those experiencing a heart attack, all the evidence suggests it is being over-utilized in stable men and women.

(Often) Unnecessary Procedures

You've no doubt noticed that a major danger in common to all of the tests is their likelihood of leading to procedures just as unnecessary as the tests themselves: namely, stent placement and bypass surgery. The evidence for this was covered in-depth in chapter 4, but it's worth one last reminder as to why these procedures are usually unnecessary.

Coronary Stent Placement

Approximately one million coronary stents will be inserted in the United States over the next year. But despite the billions of dollars that are spent on stents, the vast majority of stable patients who receive them to treat coronary blockages would have been better off being treated with lifestyle changes and medical therapy. There is no data that treating a patient's blocked coronary artery with a stent is an approach superior to managing the blockage and other unseen plaques through optimal nutrition, exercise, smoking cessation, stress reduction, and medical therapy.

By introducing a foreign object into the body, you are actually increasing the risk of clots, and the blockages that get stented are statistically unlikely to be the ones that rupture and cause heart attack. Stent placement is best reserved for the truly unstable patient, or the patient actively in the throes of a heart attack. In contrast, most stent placements in stable patients with coronary blockages wastes money and subjects the patient to added, unnecessary risk.

Coronary Artery Bypass Surgery

We perform almost a half million coronary bypass procedures each year, to the tune of billions of dollars and considerable patient risk. Bypass surgery is beneficial in select patients—those with critical left main coronary artery disease, severe triple vessel coronary artery disease and a weak heart muscle, and patients with severe disabling chest pain despite maximal medical therapy. Recommending coronary artery bypass surgery to stable patients who have a coronary blockage is inappropriate in the vast majority of cases. Remember, the largest blockages—the blockages addressed through bypass surgery—are not the ones most likely to cause a heart attack.

There have been three major studies comparing the effectiveness of coronary artery bypass surgery to that of medical therapy, and they all concluded that, with few exceptions, coronary bypass surgery neither prolonged life nor prevented heart attack compared to medical therapy.

Coronary artery bypass surgery is employed far more often than necessary: Dr. Thomas Graboys also published a study of eighty-eight patients to whom he gave a second opinion prior to recommended coronary bypass surgery. He felt that seventy-four of the eighty-eight were not candidates for surgery. Notably, all sixty patients who followed his advice and did not have surgery were alive and well years later.

Putting It All Together

Inferior doctors treat the full-blown disease. Mediocre doctors treat the disease before it becomes evident. Superior doctors prevent the disease.

—Chinese Medical Text (Huang Dee: Nai Ching), 2600 B.C.

B Y READING THIS BOOK I hope you will have gained some crucial insights regarding cardiovascular disease prevention and treatment. My bottom line regarding heart disease is this: We do far too much *intervention* in this country, and not nearly enough *prevention*. Although heart disease is the nation's number one killer, there's plenty you can do to prevent heart disease from happening to you. It requires some effort and commitment on your part, but the benefits are well worth it.

In this book I have outlined my Ten-Step Prevention Plan, which can help you prevent and even reverse heart disease. As an added benefit, you'll reduce your risk of cancer and other degenerative diseases, have more energy, feel better, and even look better. And needless to say, if you're taking steps to avoid several of the leading causes of death in America, you'll probably live longer too.

Heart disease often begins early in life, with the development of atherosclerosis. Atherosclerotic plaques build up in the linings of affected patients' arteries for decades. Aided and abetted by poor diet, lack of exercise, and ongoing low-grade inflammation, these plaques may eventually rupture, causing potentially deadly clots that can lead to heart attack and, often, death.

If atherosclerosis were unavoidable, the situation would be tragic indeed. But atherosclerosis is not unavoidable. On the contrary, it is entirely preventable. Perhaps this makes the current state of affairs in America even more tragic. The American Heart Association estimated that more than 80 *million* Americans suffered from cardiovascular disease in 2005, and more than 800,000 lives were lost to heart disease in the previous year. We're spending billions of dollars every year on surgical interventions to treat blocked coronary arteries, yet studies have repeatedly shown that, for the vast majority of patients, this has been money wasted.

Except in very specific instances, invasive cardiac care, including coronary artery bypass surgeries, angioplasties, and stent placements, *do not prolong life or prevent future heart attacks*, compared to medical therapy and lifestyle changes in stable patients with coronary artery disease. Yet hospitals and physicians continue to tout "state of the art" invasive heart treatments as the best we have to offer. We're expected to consider ourselves fortunate to live in such a scientifically and medically advanced society where high-tech procedures to address near-fatal heart disease are so readily available. We're led to believe we're fighting the good fight against an inexorable enemy. But this approach is wrong-headed and backwards. Why wait to combat this disease until after it's nearly won the battle? Why not prevent the rise of this enemy long before it becomes a formidable foe?

In a way, the American public and the cardiac intervention industry are like co-dependent addicts. Average Americans are addicted to bad dietary habits, bad lifestyle choices, and even outright laziness. Countless studies have shown the importance of a healthy diet and routine physical exercise, yet a majority of Americans largely ignore this fundamental biological requirement for the maintenance of their health. Taken together, these dietary and lifestyle choices all but guarantee heart disease.

The cardiac intervention industry, which thrives on the inevitable outcome of all this bad behavior, is a willing enabler of this toxic approach. "Don't bother to care for your own health," it seems content to say, "we'll patch you up when you get sick." To which I say, why not actively promote behavior that will prevent heart patients from becoming patients in the first place? Unfortunately, many health care providers in the cardiac intervention industry refuse to admit it's simply not a sensible or even workable solution to most heart disease.

Carefully conducted scientific studies have repeatedly shown that these invasive and expensive treatments are frequently unnecessary—just as many studies have shown that there is a better way. Ironically, the solution to coronary heart disease misery can be found in less advanced, third-world countries—where there are few, if any, advanced CAT scanners, cardiac catheterization labs, or nuclear medicine suites, but where heart attacks are infrequent.

My Vision

I've labored in the trenches of preventive cardiology for decades, and I've seen many new innovations that promised to transform the treatment of heart disease. I've also seen the tarnish form on most of these shiny new "miracle" treatments. The only approach to heart disease treatment that has never failed is prevention. "Treating" heart disease in America with prevention, rather than intervention, will require a paradigm shift, a radical reconceptualization of the way we physicians practice medicine, and in the way patients not only interact with their health care providers, but live their lives.

My vision for American medicine is this: Doctors will spend far more time *talking* with their patients, getting to know them and their problems. Doctors will spend more of their time and energy *educating* their patients about the importance of diet, exercise, and other lifestyle factors that affect cardiovascular health. In this idyllic scenario, doctors will act less out of fear of the medico-legal consequences of their actions (or inactions), and more out of concern for their patients' health. They'll treat every patient as if he or she were a member of the family rather than a number on a chart. Patients will also assume new responsibilities under this novel model for sensible health care. Patients will ask more questions of their health care providers, and they'll take more responsibility for maintaining their own health. I believe the practice of excellent medicine requires a dialogue between doctor and patient.

Doubtless, many of my colleagues will argue that this rosy scenario is an impractical pipe dream. They'll say they're already overworked, overscheduled, and underpaid, and that my suggestions are impractical at best, and naïve at worst. But consider this: If we were to implement these changes—if we were to educate our patients from a young age in how to take charge of their own lives and accept responsibility for their own health— if, in short, we were able to prevent heart disease in an entire generation, wouldn't we reap an abundance of time? We'd certainly be doing far fewer invasive cardiology procedures. And there would certainly be far more money available to invest in preventive medicine once we stopped squandering so many of our health care dollars on discredited and unnecessary invasive procedures.

Whether or not my vision for the future of American medicine ever comes to fruition in any meaningful way will depend on my fellow physicians' willingness to take a good hard look in the proverbial mirror. It also depends on you, the patient. Are you willing to take greater responsibility for your own fate? Are you willing to say no to French fries and yes to whole grains? Is the prospect of a longer, healthier life worth enough for you to put down the television remote and put on your walking shoes?

The choice is yours. To achieve my vision for a healthy America, doctors *and* patients will need to do a little soul searching. Change is never easy, and the impulse to procrastinate is often irresistible. But the status quo is clearly not working, for American patients *or* for the American health care system.

Knowledge Is Power

You've seen that medical therapy and lifestyle changes can prevent or halt the progression of coronary atherosclerosis, and even potentially reverse it. You've seen that they have been shown to help prevent heart attacks and prolong life.

You've also seen that much of the testing and surgery done today in response to heart disease is not only unnecessary but also downright dangerous to the stable patient. Angioplasty and stents don't "fix" patients. They're the equivalent of cosmetic surgery for the arteries: they may make them look good, but they don't do anything but cover up the problem. Heart bypass surgery is rarely the answer either. It doesn't do anything to change the underlying issue that created the need for surgery in the first place.

But you've also seen how you can drastically reduce your odds of developing cardiovascular disease, cancer, diabetes, hypertension, and stroke, as well as other illnesses related to unhealthy diet and lifestyle.

The Ozner Ten-Step Prevention Plan:

1. **Follow a Mediterranean Diet**. The Mediterranean diet has been consumed by the people of the Mediterranean

basin for thousands of years, and is the only diet that has ever received so much scientific scrutiny and validation: carefully documented scientific research conducted over the past six decades has conclusively proven that this diet drastically reduces your risk of cardiovascular disease. It's also the basis for the diet I have successfully used in my preventive cardiology practice for over twenty years. It features vegetables, fruits, whole grains, legumes, nuts, red wine, minimal lean meat, extra virgin olive oil as the primary source of fat, plenty of fish, and ideally, no processed foods, refined carbohydrates, or trans fats.

2. **Exercise Regularly**. Studies show that exercise doesn't have to be excessive, and it doesn't even have to take place all at once, but one way or another, you need to get at least thirty minutes of it daily to maintain optimum cardiovascular health. Forget the excuses. It doesn't require an expensive gym membership (although gym memberships are fine, if used) or an investment in bulky or expensive exercise equipment. A simple pair of comfortable walking shoes should be sufficient to start you on the road to more energy and better health.

3. **Manage Your Stress**. Relentless stress is toxic to the mind and body. Take time to invest in relaxation. Practice yoga or tai chi, take anger management classes, laugh it up with friends, practice meditation, or find a relaxing and engaging hobby. Do whatever it takes to catch your breath, calm down, and disconnect from the hustle and bustle of your busy life on a routine basis. The world won't come to an end if you do. And if you don't, *you* may well come to an abrupt end.

4. **Take Command of Your Blood Pressure**. Monitor and control your blood pressure. Follow a diet and lifestyle that keeps your blood vessels flexible, and your blood pressure below 120/80 mmHg.

5. **Control Your Cholesterol**. Monitor and control your cholesterol level. Follow a diet and lifestyle that keeps HDL cholesterol high and LDL cholesterol and triglycerides low.

6. **Reduce Free Radicals and Oxidative Stress**. There is a war going on in your body between free radicals and antioxidants. Fight free radicals, and the oxidative stress and disease that results, by giving your body's natural antioxidants plenty of reinforcements in the form of fresh fruits and vegetables. Avoid toxins, including cigarette smoke, to keep free radical production as low as possible.

7. **Avoid Chronic Inflammation**. Control inflammation by following the anti-inflammatory Miami Mediterranean diet and consuming plenty of omega-3 fatty acids in the form of cold water fish, and certain vegetable and grain sources. Proper dental hygiene and regular dental cleaning and check-ups help to guard against a frequent cause of chronic inflammation, chronic periodontal disease. Treating other conditions that lead to chronic inflammation, such as chronic bronchitis, prostatitis, and arthritis, also helps to quell the fires of inflammation.

8. **Prevent Metabolic Syndrome and Diabetes**. Prevent and reverse metabolic syndrome and its frequent end result, type 2 diabetes, by following prudent diet and lifestyle recommendations.

9. **Have an Annual Physical Exam with Comprehensive Lab**. An ongoing relationship with your personal treating physician is important. Have an annual physical exam and discuss prevention strategies with your doctor—even if you are healthy and feel well. In addition, have an advanced lipid profile done. Specifically, make sure your doctor tests for three things: particle number, hs-CRP, and LP(a). These laboratory tests provide great-

er insight into the specific cardiovascular disease risk factors that may impact your individual situation.

10. **Avoid Unnecessary Diagnostic Tests and Procedures**. Routine cardiovascular screening with CAT scans are not recommended for healthy people— they are expensive (and not covered by insurance), and they deliver a significant dose of ionizing radiation that may increase the risk of cancer. Nuclear stress tests also result in radiation exposure and can usually be replaced by a stress echo (ultrasound) study. Cardiac catheterization is not always as safe or simple a procedure as you may be led to believe. Since it often leads to simultaneous procedures, such as balloon angioplasty and/or stent placement, you may end up with far more than you bargained for. Don't let yourself be talked into coronary bypass surgery unless it's truly indicated. Seriously weigh the pros and cons before submitting to any of these procedures. And do not hesitate to seek a second opinion if your physician is unwilling to discuss risks, benefits, and alternatives.

You can prevent, halt, or even reverse heart disease. The choice to do so is up to you.

National Cholesterol Guidelines and Coronary Heart Disease Risk Assessment

ATP III At-A-Glance

Detection, Evaluation, and Treatment of High Blood Cholesterol in Adults (Reprinted with Permission of the National Cholesterol Education Program)

TABLE OF CONTENTS

STEP 6: Initiate therapeutic lifestyle changes (TLC) if LDL is above goal

STEP 7: Consider adding drug therapy if LDL exceeds levels shown in Step 5 table

STEP 8: Identify metabolic syndrome and treat, if present, after 3 months of TLC

STEP 9: Treat elevated triglycerides

STEP 1: Determine lipoprotein levels—obtain complete lipoprotein profile after 9- to 12-hour fast.

ATP III Classification of LDL, Total, and HDL Cholesterol (mg/dL)

LDL Cholesterol - Primary Target of Therapy

<100	Optimal
100–129	Near Optimal/Above Optimal
130–159	Borderline High
160–189	High
≥190	Very high

Total Cholesterol

<200	Desirable
200–239	Borderline High
≥240	High

HDL Cholesterol

<40	Low
≥60	High

STEP 2: Identify presence of clinical atherosclerotic disease that confers high risk for coronary heart disease (CHD) events (CHD risk equivalent).

- Clinical CHD
- Symptomatic carotid artery disease
- Peripheral arterial disease
- Abdominal aortic aneurysm

STEP 3: Determine presence of major risk factors (other than LDL).

Major Risk Factors (Exclusive of LDL Cholesterol) That Modify LDL Goals
- Cigarette smoking
- Hypertension (BP ≥140/90 mmHg or on antihypertensive medication)
- Low HDL cholesterol (<40 mg/dl)*
- Family history of premature CHD (CHD in male first degree relative <55 years; CHD in female first degree relative <65 years)
- Age (men ≥45 years; women ≥55 years)

* HDL cholesterol ≥60 mg/dL counts as a "negative" risk factor; its presence removes one risk factor from the total count.

NOTE: In ATP III, diabetes is regarded as a CHD risk equivalent.

STEP 4: If 2+ risk factors (other than LDL) are present without CHD or CHD risk equivalent, assess 10-year (short-term) CHD risk (see Framingham tables).

Three levels of 10-year risk:
- >20% (CHD risk equivalent)
- 10-20%
- <10%

STEP 5: Determine risk category.

Establish LDL goal of therapy
- Determine need for therapeutic lifestyle changes (TLC)
- Determine level for drug consideration
- LDL cholesterol goals and cutpoints for therapeutic lifestyle changes (TLC) and drug therapy in different risk categories

Risk Category	LDL Goal	LDL Level at Which to Initiate Therapeutic Lifestyle Changes (TLC)	LDL Level at Which to Consider Drug Therapy
CHD or CHD Risk Equivalents (10-year risk >20%)	<100 mg/dL	≥100 mg/dL	≥130 mg/dL (100-129 mg/dL: drug optional)*
2+ Risk Factors (10-year risk ≤20%)	<130 mg/dL	≥130 mg/dL	10-year risk 10-20%: ≥130 mg/dL 10-year risk <10%: ≥160 mg/dL
0-1 Risk Factor**	<160 mg/dL	≥160 mg/dL	≥190 mg/dL (160-189 mg/dL: LDL-lowering drug optional)

* Some authorities recommend use of LDL-lowering drugs in this category if an LDL cholesterol <100 mg/dL cannot be achieved by therapeutic lifestyle changes. Others prefer use of drugs that primarily modify triglycerides and HDL, e.g., nicotinic acid or fibrate. Clinical judgment also may call for deferring drug therapy in this subcategory.

** Almost all people with 0-1 risk factor have a 10-year risk <10%, thus 10-year risk assessment in people with 0-1 risk factor is not necessary.

STEP 6: Initiate therapeutic lifestyle changes (TLC) if LDL is above goal.

TLC Features
- TLC Diet:
  - Saturated fat <7% of calories, cholesterol <200 mg/day
  - Consider increased viscous (soluble) fiber (10–25 g/day) and plant stanols/sterols (2g/day) as therapeutic options to enhance LDL lowering
- Weight management
- Increased physical activity

STEP 7: Consider adding drug therapy if LDL exceeds levels shown in Step 5 table.

- Consider drug simultaneously with TLC for CHD and CHD equivalents.

- Consider adding drug to TLC after 3 months for other risk categories.

Drugs Affecting Lipoprotein Metabolism

Drug Class	Agents and Daily Doses	Lipid/Lipoprotein Effects	Side Effects	Contraindications
HMG CoA reductase inhibitors (statins)	Lovastatin (20-80 mg), Pravastatin (20-40 mg), Simvastatin (20-80 mg), Fluvastatin (20-80 mg), Atorvastatin (10-80 mg), Cerivastatin (0.4-0.8 mg)	LDL-C ⇩18-55% HDL-C ⇧5-15% TG ⇩7-30%	Myopathy Increased liver enzymes	Absolute: - Active or chronic liver disease Relative: - Concomitant use of certain drugs*
Bile acid Sequestrants	Cholestyramine (4-16 g) Colestipol (5-20 g) Colesevelam (2.6-3.8 g)	LDL-C ⇩15-30% HDL-C ⇧3-5% TG No change or increase	Gastrointestinal distress Constipation Decreased absorption of other drugs	Absolute: - dysbeta-lipoproteinemia - TG >400 mg/dL Relative: - TG >200 mg/dL
Nicotinic acid	Immediate release (crystalline) nicotinic acid (1.5-3 gm), extended release nicotinic acid (Niaspan ®) (1-2 g), sustained release nicotinic acid (1-2 g)	LDL-C ⇩5-25% HDL-C ⇧15-35% TG ⇩20-50%	Flushing Hyperglycemia Hyperuricemia (or gout) Upper GI distress Hepatotoxicity	Absolute: - Chronic liver disease - Severe gout Relative: - Diabetes - Hyperuricemia - Peptic ulcer disease
Fibric acids	Gemfibrozil (600 mg BID) Fenofibrate (200 mg) Clofibrate (1000 mg BID)	LDL-C ⇩5-20% (may be increased in patients with high TG) HDL-C ⇧10-20% TG ⇩20-50%	Dyspepsia Gallstones Myopathy	Absolute: - Severe renal disease - Severe hepatic disease

* Cyclosporine, macrolide antibiotics, various anti-fungal agents, and cytochrome P-450 inhibitors (fibrates and niacin should be used with appropriate caution).

STEP 8: Identify metabolic syndrome and treat, if present, after 3 months of TLC.

Clinical Identification of Metabolic Syndrome—Any 3 of the Following:

Risk Factor	Defining Level
Abdominal obesity*	Waist circumference**
Men	>102 cm (>40 in)
Women	>88 cm (>35 in)
Triglycerides	≥150 mg/dL
HDL cholesterol	
Men	<40 mg/dl
Women	<50 mg/dl
blood pressure	≥130/≥85 mmHg
Fasting glucose	≥110 mg/dL

* Overweight and obesity are associated with insulin resistance and metabolic syndrome. However, the presence of abdominal obesity is more highly correlated with metabolic risk factors than is an elevated body mass index (BMI). Therefore, the simple measure of waist circumference is recommended to identify the body weight component of metabolic syndrome.

** Some male patients can develop multiple metabolic risk factors when the waist circumference is only marginally increased, e.g., 94-102 cm (37-39 in). Such patients may have a strong genetic contribution to insulin resistance. They should benefit from changes in life habits, similarly to men with categorical increases in waist circumference.

Treatment of Metabolic Syndrome

- Treat underlying causes (overweight/obesity and physical inactivity):
  - Intensify weight management
  - Increase physical activity
- Treat lipid and non-lipid risk factors if they persist despite these lifestyle therapies:
  - Treat hypertension
  - Use aspirin for CHD patients to reduce prothrombotic state
  - Treat elevated triglycerides and/or low HDL (as shown in Step 9 below)

STEP 9: Treat elevated triglycerides.

ATP III Classification of Serum Triglycerides (mg/dL)

< 150	Normal
150–199	Borderline high
200-499	High
≥500	Very high

Treatment of Elevated Triglycerides (≥150 mg/dL)
- Primary aim of therapy is to reach LDL goal
- Intensify weight management
- Increase physical activity
- If triglycerides are ≥200 mg/dL after LDL goal is reached, set secondary goal for non-HDL cholesterol (total - HDL) 30 mg/dL higher than LDL goal

Comparison of LDL Cholesterol and Non-HDL Cholesterol Goals for Three Risk Categories=

Risk Category	LDL Goal (mg/dL)	Non-HDL Goal (mg/dL)
CHD and CHD Risk Equivalent (10-year risk for CHD >20%)	<100	<130
Multiple (2+) Risk Factors and 10-year risk ≤20%	<130	<160
0-1 Risk Factor	<160	<190

If triglycerides 200–499 mg/dL after LDL goal is reached, consider adding drug if needed to reach non-HDL goal:
- Intensify therapy with LDL-lowering drug, or
- Add nicotinic acid or fibrate to further lower VLDL

If triglycerides ≥500 mg/dL, first lower triglycerides to prevent pancreatitis:
- Very low-fat diet (≤15% of calories from fat)
- Weight management and physical activity
- Fibrate or nicotinic acid

- When triglycerides <500 mg/dL, turn to LDL-lowering therapy

Treatment of low HDL cholesterol (<40 mg/dL)
- First reach LDL goal, then:
- Intensify weight management and increase physical activity
- If triglycerides 200–499 mg/dL, achieve non-HDL goal
- If triglycerides <200 mg/dL (isolated low HDL) in CHD or CHD equivalent, consider nicotinic acid or fibrate

---

U.S. DEPARTMENT OF HEALTH AND HUMAN SERVICES
Public Health Service
National Institutes of Health
National Heart, Lung, and Blood Institute
NIH Publication No. 01-3305
May 2001

APPENDIX B

Cellular Respiration and Free Radical Production

WHEN WE THINK OF RESPIRATION, we think of the ordinarily automatic process of breathing. The muscles of the rib cage and diaphragm work to expand the lungs, which take in several liters of air, about one-fifth of which is composed of oxygen atoms. Atmospheric oxygen is actually in a form known as molecular oxygen. It's composed of two oxygen atoms in a tight embrace. Once oxygen-bearing air rushes deep into the recesses of the lungs, tiny sacs called alveoli extract the precious gas, which is then transported across the delicate membranes of the alveoli and enters the bloodstream. (Waste gas—carbon dioxide—is expelled from the bloodstream and exhaled in roughly the reverse of this process.)

After it is delivered to the heart and pumped to the farthest reaches of the body, oxygen-enriched blood delivers its precious cargo to individual cells, which need it to extract energy from glucose and other nutrients. The demand of different types of cells and tissues for energy and oxygen varies. Brain cells' requirement for energy, and thus for glucose and oxygen, is prodigious. The same is true of muscle cells, especially muscle cells that are working hard. This is why the brain is among the first organs to die when deprived of oxygen. It is also why we breathe more deeply and more rapidly while exercising; working muscles burn fuel rapidly. Since it never rests, the heart muscle is especially vulnerable to any interruption in its supply of well-oxygenated blood and this is why heart attacks may be fatal.

When we are hungry, we know we're running low on fuel, and we consume food for energy. Almost immediately, we feel better—more energetic. But releasing the inherent energy stored in our food is not quite as simple as just eating an apple. A complex process of digestion must take place first. Suffice it to say that eventually most food is converted to its simplest components (though some components are too difficult to break down sufficiently, and so are eliminated). Carbohydrates are broken down into simple sugar molecules, in the form of glucose. These are ushered into individual cells by insulin molecules. Cells also make use of amino acids, the building blocks of proteins, as well as fatty acids, derived from various fats and oils.

But even glucose—a simple molecule composed of just six carbon atoms, with a handful of hydrogen and oxygen atoms attached—is not yet in a form that will allow the body to take advantage of the energy it contains. To do so, the molecule requires further "processing." This processing takes the form of numerous chemical reactions, also known as metabolic pathways. Taken together, all these metabolic pathways are known as *cellular respiration* (also called aerobic respiration). The first is *glycolysis,* followed by *pyruvate decarboxylation,* then the *Krebs cycle,* and finally, *oxidative phosphorylation,* or the *electron transport chain.* Glycolysis, which takes place within the cytoplasm (the liquid, interior portion) of a given cell, involves the metabolism, or chemical conversion, of a glucose molecule into another type of molecule, a *pyruvate* molecule. A small amount of energy is released by this conversion, but the majority of the original energy stored in the glucose molecule is still contained within the newly formed pyruvate molecule. To release it, the pyruvate molecule is shuttled to the interior of a tiny organelle within the cell called a *mitochondrion*.

Mitochondria range in number from a handful to hundreds per cell, depending on a given cell's demand for energy. Muscle cells, for example, are crowded with many hundreds of these organelles, and liver cells may contain 2,000 or more, while red blood cells have none. Mitochondria are often referred to as the "powerhouses" of the cells because of their role in extracting energy from pyruvate molecules. A specific metabolic pathway, known as the Krebs cycle (or citric acid cycle), uses oxygen to convert pyruvate, through oxidation, into the ultimate energy "coin of the realm," *adenosine triphosphate*, or ATP. This happens through a series of electron transfers known as the *electron transport chain*. This step relies on various enzymes, including coenzyme Q10, or CoQ10.

Cellular respiration is relatively efficient, releasing roughly 40 percent of the energy stored in a given glucose molecule. While this may sound wasteful, the most common biochemical alternative is achieved through a process known as anaerobic respiration— essentially a fermentation reaction, in which pyruvate is converted (in skeletal muscle cells, for example) to lactic acid and two ATP molecules. Considerable energy remains locked up in the lactic acid molecules, which means this form of respiration is far less efficient.

Of course, when we say the Krebs cycle, and subsequent electron transport chain, is relatively efficient, the operative term is "relatively." There is occasionally some leakage of high-energy electrons from the electron transport chain, and these stray electrons quickly react with oxygen molecules to generate small, highly reactive molecules called *reactive oxygen species* (ROS)—which include *free radicals* like oxygen ions and peroxides. Although some ROS are occasionally used by cells as signaling agents, for the most part these reactive molecules are problematic. One of the most dangerous of these is *superoxide anion,* or simply *superoxide.*

Superoxide is so toxic that the immune system actually harnesses it for use as a weapon to kill invading pathogens. But when superoxide is generated accidentally, it becomes a rogue ROS. These ROS molecules are what is responsible for oxidative stress, a state of imbalance in which the body's antioxidants are overwhelmed by ROS. Under these conditions, ROS are dangerous because they contain unpaired electrons that desperately "want" to pair with other electrons. And they don't care where these partners come from. In their rush to kidnap electrons from any available source, they may damage proteins, lipids, and even DNA. And as these free radicals steal electrons they create new free radicals and an ongoing chain reaction begins.

Unfortunately, unless these free radicals are rapidly neutralized by the body's native antioxidant resources, or by antioxidant molecules obtained through the diet—which provide free radicals with an extra electron without becoming free radicals themselves—their theft of electrons from other molecules tends to cripple those molecules, initiating a cycle of cellular, and eventually tissue, degradation that results in disease.

Selected Recipes and Menu Plan from *The Miami Mediterranean Diet*

This sample 7-day menu plan, with recipes drawn from *The Miami Mediterranean Diet*, will help get you started on your way to losing weight and lowering your risk of heart disease. For more recipes like these and an extended 14-day menu plan, check out *The Miami Mediterranean Diet*.

7-Day Menu Plan

DAY 1

BREAKFAST

    4 ounces vegetable or fruit juice
    1 slice whole wheat toast with extra-virgin olive oil or 1 teaspoon vegetable spread (trans fat–free canola/olive oil spread)
    1 teaspoon jam
    ½ cup plain low-fat yogurt (sweetened with non-caloric sweetener if desired)
    ½ cup blueberries or strawberries
    8 ounces water

Coffee or tea (soy or non-fat milk, trans fat–free coffee creamer, and non-caloric sweetener if desired)

- APPROX. 239 CALORIES

Optional Midmorning Snack

10–20 almonds or walnuts
8 ounces water or non-caloric beverage

LUNCH

Chickpea Pita Pocket (page 214)
1 medium apple, sliced and drizzled with honey
8 ounces water or non-caloric beverage

- APPROX. 319 CALORIES

Optional Midday Snack

10–20 almonds or walnuts
8 ounces water or non-caloric beverage

DINNER

1 jumbo clove Roasted Garlic (page 205)
½ (6-inch) whole wheat pita loaf, split open, sprayed with olive oil and herb seasonings of choice, and toasted in the microwave or oven until crispy
Goat Cheese Stuffed Tomato (page 205)
Linguine and Mixed Seafood (page 216)
Fresh vegetable of choice (flavor with olive oil or vegetable spread as desired)
Drunken Apricots (page 224)
8 ounces water
1 or 2 (4-ounce) glasses of red wine or purple grape juice
Coffee or tea (soy or non-fat milk, trans fat–free coffee creamer, and non-caloric sweetener if desired)

- APPROX. 761 CALORIES

Optional Evening Snack

1 apple or orange
8 ounces water

DAY 2

BREAKFAST

4 ounces vegetable or fruit juice

½ cup egg whites with diced onions, tomato, and green bell peppers
cooked into an omelet

1 slice whole wheat toast with extra-virgin olive oil or 1 teaspoon
vegetable spread (trans fat–free canola/olive oil spread)

1 teaspoon fruit jam

½ small banana

8 ounces water

Coffee or tea (soy or non-fat milk, trans fat–free coffee creamer, and
non-caloric sweetener if desired)

- APPROX. 230 CALORIES

Optional Midmorning Snack

10–20 almonds or walnuts

8 ounces water or non-caloric beverage

LUNCH

Greek Olive and Feta Cheese Pasta Salad (page 206)

½ (6-inch) whole wheat pita loaf, toasted if desired

⅛-inch fresh cantaloupe

8 ounces water or non-caloric beverage

- APPROX. 354 CALORIES

Optional Midday Snack

1 apple

8 ounces water or non-caloric beverage

DINNER

1 jumbo clove Roasted Garlic (page 205)

½ (6-inch) whole wheat pita loaf, split open, sprayed with olive oil
and herb seasonings of choice, and toasted until crispy in the oven
or microwave

6–8 marinated assorted olives

Grilled Citrus Salmon with Garlic Greens (page 217)

Grilled Eggplant (page 222)
Strawberries and Balsamic Syrup (page 225)
8 ounces water
1 or 2 (4-ounce) glasses of red wine or purple grape juice
Coffee or tea (soy or non-fat milk, trans fat–free coffee creamer, and
non-caloric sweetener if desired)

- APPROX. 653 CALORIES

Optional Evening Snack

1 apple or orange
8 ounces water

DAY 3

BREAKFAST

4 ounces vegetable or fruit juice
½ cup egg whites with diced onions, tomato, and green bell peppers
1 slice whole wheat toast with olive oil (extra-virgin) or 1 teaspoon
vegetable spread (trans fat–free canola/olive oil spread)
1 teaspoon fruit jam
1 medium fresh peach or 1 large plum
8 ounces water
Coffee or tea (soy or non-fat milk, trans fat–free coffee creamer, and
non-caloric sweetener if desired)

- APPROX. 230 CALORIES

Optional Midmorning Snack

10–20 almonds or walnuts
8 ounces water or non-caloric beverage

LUNCH

Italian Minestrone Soup with Pesto (page 209)
1 slice whole grain crusty bread with extra-virgin olive oil
½ cup fresh raspberries
½ cup plain low-fat yogurt, sweetened with non-caloric sweetener if
desired
8 ounces water or non-caloric beverage

- APPROX. 390 CALORIES

Optional Midday Snack

1 apple
8 ounces water or non-caloric beverage

DINNER

Simple Spanish Salad (page 207)
1 jumbo clove Roasted Garlic (page 205)
½ (6-inch) whole wheat pita loaf, split open, sprayed with olive oil
  and herb seasonings of choice, and toasted until crispy in the oven
  or microwave
1 slice soft goat cheese
6–8 marinated mixed olives
Fresh vegetable of choice (flavor with olive oil or vegetable spread as
  desired)
Chicken Piccata (page 218)
Honeydew Sorbet (page 225)
8 ounces water
1 or 2 (4-ounce) glasses of red wine or purple grape juice
Coffee or tea (soy or non-fat milk, trans fat–free coffee creamer, and
  non-caloric sweetener if desired)

* APPROX. 725 CALORIES

Optional Evening Snack

2 Meringue Cookies (page 226)
Green tea or 8 ounces water

DAY 4

BREAKFAST

4 ounces vegetable or fruit juice
2 slices whole wheat toast
2 tablespoons fresh chunky peanut butter
2 teaspoons honey
½ ruby red grapefruit, sweetened with non-caloric sweetener if
  desired
8 ounces water
Coffee or tea (soy or non-fat milk, trans fat–free coffee creamer, and
  non-caloric sweetener if desired)

* APPROX. 385 CALORIES

Optional Midmorning Snack

10–20 almonds or walnuts
8 ounces water or non-caloric beverage

LUNCH

Light Caesar Salad (page 207)
1 slice Pizza Margherita (page 213)
10–20 seedless grapes
8 ounces water or non-caloric beverage

• APPROX. 302 CALORIES

Optional Midday Snack

1 apple
8 ounces water or non-caloric beverage

DINNER

1 clove jumbo Roasted Garlic (page 205)
½ (6-inch) whole wheat pita loaf, split open, sprayed with extra-virgin olive oil and herb seasonings of choice, and toasted until crispy in the oven or microwave
Chilly Tomato Soup (page 210)
Fennel Salad (page 208)
Fresh vegetable of choice (flavor with olive oil or vegetable spread as desired)
Spicy Whole Wheat Capellini with Garlic (page 219)
8 ounces water
Sweet Plum Compote (page 227)
1 or 2 (4-ounce) glasses of red wine or purple grape juice
Coffee or tea (soy or non-fat milk, trans fat–free coffee creamer, and non-caloric sweetener if desired)

• APPROX. 786 CALORIES

Optional Evening Snack

1 apple or orange
8 ounces water

DAY 5

BREAKFAST

4 ounces vegetable or fruit juice

1 slice whole wheat toast with extra-virgin olive oil or 1 teaspoon vegetable spread (trans fat–free canola/olive oil spread)

1 teaspoon fruit jam

½ cup plain low-fat yogurt, sweetened with non-caloric sweetener if desired

½ cup blueberries or strawberries

8 ounces water

Coffee or tea (soy or non-fat milk, trans fat–free coffee creamer, and non-caloric sweetener if desired)

- APPROX. 289 CALORIES

Optional Midmorning Snack

10–20 almonds or walnuts

8 ounces water or non-caloric beverage

LUNCH

Hearty Bean Soup (page 211)

1 slice whole grain bread with extra-virgin olive oil or 1 teaspoon vegetable spread (trans fat–free canola/olive oil spread)

3 fresh apricots

8 ounces water or non-caloric beverage

- APPROX. 414 CALORIES

Optional Midday Snack

1 apple

8 ounces water or non-caloric beverage

DINNER

4 tablespoons hummus

½ (6-inch) whole wheat pita loaf, split open, sprayed with extra-virgin olive oil and herb seasonings of choice, and toasted until crispy in the oven or microwave

4 tomato wedges topped with slivers of red onion, freshly grated mozzarella cheese, chopped fresh cilantro, and drizzled with aged balsamic vinegar and 1 teaspoon extra-virgin olive oil

Fettuccine with Smoked Salmon and Basil Pesto (page 219)
Peach Marsala Compote (page 227)
1 or 2 (4-ounce) glasses of red wine or purple grape juice
8 ounces water
Coffee or tea (soy or non-fat milk, trans fat–free coffee creamer, and non-caloric sweetener if desired)

• APPROX. 774 CALORIES

Optional Evening Snack

2 Meringue Cookies (page 226)
Green tea or 8 ounces water

DAY 6

BREAKFAST

4 ounces vegetable or fruit juice
½ cup dry oatmeal, cooked and sweetened with non-caloric sweetener if desired
1 tablespoon seedless black raisins
1 medium orange, sliced
8 ounces water
Coffee or tea (soy or non-fat milk, trans fat–free coffee creamer, and non-caloric sweetener if desired)

• APPROX. 292 CALORIES

Optional Midmorning Snack

10–20 almonds or walnuts
8 ounces water or non-caloric beverage

LUNCH

Veggie Wrap (page 215)
Roasted Peppers (page 222)
6–8 marinated mixed olives
1 medium fresh pear, peach, or apple
8 ounces water or non-caloric beverage

• APPROX. 601 CALORIES

Optional Midday Snack
1 apple
8 ounces water or non-caloric beverage

DINNER
1 jumbo clove Roasted Garlic (page 205)
½ (6-inch) whole wheat pita loaf, split open, sprayed with olive oil and herb seasonings, and toasted until crispy in the oven or microwave
Mediterranean Mixed Greens (page 208)
Baked Tilapia (page 220)
Classic Spinach and Pine Nuts (page 223)
Strawberries Amaretto (page 228)
8 ounces water
1 or 2 (4-ounce) glasses of red wine or purple grape juice
Coffee or tea (soy or non-fat milk, trans fat–free coffee creamer, and non-caloric sweetener if desired)

- APPROX. 597 CALORIES

Optional Evening Snack
2 Meringue Cookies (page 226)
Green tea or 8 ounces water

DAY 7

BREAKFAST
4 ounces vegetable or fruit juice
½ cup egg whites with diced red onion, tomato, and green bell peppers cooked into an omelet
1 slice whole wheat toast with extra-virgin olive oil or 1 teaspoon vegetable spread (trans fat–free canola/olive oil spread)
1 teaspoon fruit jam
1 purple plum
8 ounces water
Coffee or tea (soy or non-fat milk, trans fat–free coffee creamer, and non-caloric sweetener if desired)

- APPROX. 230 CALORIES

Optional Midmorning Snack

10–20 almonds or walnuts
8 ounces water or non-caloric beverage

LUNCH

Eggplant Soup (page 212)
1 slice whole grain crusty bread, drizzled with extra-virgin olive oil
and herb seasonings of choice
1 large kiwi fruit, sliced
½ cup fresh strawberries, sliced
8 ounces water or non-caloric beverage

- APPROX. 420 CALORIES

Optional Midday Snack

1 apple
8 ounces water or non-caloric beverage

DINNER

1 slice whole grain bread with extra-virgin olive oil and herb
seasonings of choice
6–8 marinated assorted olives
Broccoli with Fresh Garlic (page 224)
Fettuccine with Sundried Tomatoes and Goat Cheese (page 221)
Fresh Fruit Kabobs and Cinnamon Honey Dip (page 228)
8 ounces water
1 or 2 (4-ounce) glasses of red wine or purple grape juice
Coffee or tea (soy or non-fat milk, trans fat–free coffee creamer, and
non-caloric sweetener if desired)

- APPROX. 1050 CALORIES

Optional Evening Snack

1 apple or orange
8 ounces water

Appetizers

ROASTED GARLIC

(MAKES 4–5 SERVINGS)

1 elephant jumbo garlic head
Extra-virgin olive oil to drizzle
Dry seasonings of choice (optional)

Holding entire head of garlic, cut off the top leaf points of each clove to expose a small portion of the clove. Keep the remainder of leaves intact around the body of the garlic head. Place trimmed garlic head in a tight-fitting oven-safe bowl, trimmed side up. Drizzle a small amount of olive oil over the top of the head and down around the sides. Sprinkle with your favorite seasoning (optional). Place garlic on middle rack of oven and bake at 400 degrees for 20–30 minutes, or until cloves are soft and a light golden brown. Remove from oven and spread garlic on crusty bread, or add to vegetables, omelets, or pasta.

Approx. 59 calories per serving
3g protein, 0.2g total fat, <1g saturated fat, 0 trans fat,
13g carbohydrates, 0 cholesterol, 7mg sodium, 1g fiber

Salads

GOAT CHEESE STUFFED TOMATOES

(MAKES 2 SERVINGS)

6–8 leaves arugula
2 medium ripe tomatoes
3 ounces crumbled feta cheese
Salt and pepper to taste
Balsamic vinegar
Extra-virgin olive oil
Red onion, very thinly sliced
Fresh chopped parsley

Place 3–4 leaves arugula in the center of each salad plate. Cut tops (about ¼ inch) off the tomatoes. With a paring knife, core out the center of the tomatoes, about ½ inch deep. Fill tomatoes with crumbled feta cheese, add salt and pepper to taste, and drizzle with balsamic vinegar and extra-virgin olive oil. Garnish with red onion slices and chopped parsley. Serve at room temperature.

Approx. 142 calories per serving
7g protein, 13g total fat, 3g saturated fat, 0 trans fat,
7g carbohydrates, 37mg cholesterol, 485mg sodium, 1g fiber

GREEK OLIVE AND FETA CHEESE PASTA
(MAKES 4 SERVINGS)

4½ ounces ziti pasta
3 ounces crumbled feta cheese
10 small Greek olives, pitted and coarsely chopped
¼ cup fresh, coarsely chopped basil leaves
2 cloves garlic, finely minced
1 tablespoon extra-virgin olive oil
¼ teaspoon finely chopped hot pepper
½ red bell pepper, diced
½ yellow bell pepper, diced
2 plum tomatoes, seeded and diced

Bring water to a boil, add pasta, and cook pasta until *al dente*. Remove from heat, drain pasta, and return to pot, drizzling with scant amount of olive oil to keep pasta from sticking together. Set aside. In a large serving bowl combine feta cheese, olives, basil, garlic, olive oil, and hot peppers, then set aside for 30 minutes. Add cooked pasta, red and yellow bell peppers, and tomato; toss ingredients well. Cover and refrigerate for at least 1 hour, until well chilled. Toss again before serving.

This salad goes well as a side dish to grilled lamb or fish.

Approx. 235 calories per serving
7g protein, 10g total fat, 1g saturated fat, 0 trans fat,
27g carbohydrates, 18mg cholesterol, 98mg sodium, 2g fiber

SIMPLE SPANISH SALAD
(MAKES 6 SERVINGS)

1 bag (2 bunches) cleaned and trimmed romaine lettuce, torn into
  bite-sized pieces
3 medium ripe tomatoes cut into ¼-inch wedges
1 large sweet onion, thinly sliced
1 green bell pepper, seeded and thinly sliced
1 red bell pepper, seeded and thinly sliced
¼ cup chopped and pitted marinated green olives
¼ cup chopped and pitted black olives
¼ cup extra-virgin olive oil
3 tablespoons balsamic vinegar
Salt and freshly ground pepper to taste

Place a bed of romaine lettuce on six chilled salad plates. Arrange
tomatoes, onions, peppers, and olives on top of the lettuce on each
plate. Mix olive oil and vinegar together; drizzle over salad. Add salt
and pepper if desired and serve.

Approx. 107 calories per serving
2g protein, 9g total fat, 1g saturated fat, 0 trans fat,
7g carbohydrates, 0 cholesterol, 145mg sodium, 3g fiber

LIGHT CAESAR SALAD
(MAKES 6 SERVINGS)

1–2 bunches packaged pre-cleaned romaine lettuce, torn in pieces
½ cup non-fat plain yogurt
2 teaspoons lemon juice
2½ teaspoons balsamic vinegar
1 teaspoon Worcestershire sauce
2 cloves freshly minced garlic
½ teaspoon anchovy paste
½ cup grated Parmesan cheese
10 small pitted black olives, chopped

Clean and pat dry romaine lettuce and place in large salad bowl.
In a blender mix yogurt, lemon juice, vinegar, Worcestershire sauce,

garlic, anchovy paste, and ¼ cup Parmesan cheese until smooth. Pour mixture over lettuce and toss. Garnish with remaining cheese and olives.

Approx. 49 calories per serving
4g protein, 1g total fat, <0.1g saturated fat, 0 trans fat,
4g carbohydrates, 4mg cholesterol, 112mg sodium, 1g fiber

FENNEL SALAD
(MAKES 4–6 SERVINGS)

1 large clove garlic, halved
1 large fennel bulb, thinly sliced
½ English cucumber, thinly sliced
1 tablespoon minced fresh chives
8 large radishes, thinly sliced
3 tablespoons extra-virgin olive oil
2½ tablespoons freshly squeezed lemon juice
Salt and freshly ground pepper to taste
Marinated mixed olives (optional)

Rub the inside of a large bowl with garlic. Add fennel, cucumber, chives, and radishes. In a separate bowl whisk together olive oil, fresh lemon juice, and salt and pepper to taste. Pour olive oil mixture over salad and toss to mix. Garnish with marinated olives if desired.

Approx. 76 calories per serving
0 protein, 10g total fat, 1g saturated fat, 0 trans fat,
3g carbohydrates, 2mg cholesterol, 20mg sodium, 1g fiber

MEDITERRANEAN MIXED GREENS
(MAKES 4–6 SERVINGS)

6 cups assorted fresh mixed greens (such as arugula, radicchio, baby
    spinach, watercress, and romaine)
1 small red onion, thinly sliced and separated into rings
20 firm cherry tomatoes, halved
¼ cup chopped walnuts
¼ cup dried cranberries

For Dressing:

2 tablespoons balsamic vinegar
4 tablespoons extra-virgin olive oil
1 tablespoon water
½ teaspoon crushed dried oregano
2 cloves garlic, finely minced
Crumbled feta cheese (optional)
Freshly ground pepper to taste

In a large salad bowl, combine greens, onion, tomatoes, walnuts, and cranberries. Gently toss.

Dressing:

Combine vinegar, oil, water, oregano, and garlic; shake well. Pour dressing over salad and toss lightly to coat. Garnish with feta cheese, if desired, and fresh pepper.

Approx. 140 calories per serving
2g protein, 12g total fat, 1g saturated fat, 0 trans fat,
6g carbohydrates, 0 cholesterol, 47mg sodium, 1g fiber

Soups

ITALIAN MINESTRONE SOUP WITH PESTO
(MAKES 6–8 SERVINGS)

1 cup dried cannellini beans
4 cups low-sodium, fat-free chicken broth
4 cups water
2 medium white potatoes, peeled and diced
2 ounces dry ditalini pasta
2 large carrots, chopped
3 stalks celery, chopped
½ cup chopped white onion
2 cloves garlic, minced
1 cup tomato juice
3 plum tomatoes, chopped

1 large zucchini, chopped
Freshly shredded Parmesan cheese for garnish (optional)

For pesto:

1 cup fresh basil leaves
1 teaspoon crumbled dried basil leaves
4 cloves garlic, finely minced
3 tablespoons extra-virgin olive oil
½ cup grated Parmesan cheese
Salt and freshly ground pepper to taste

Rinse dried cannellini beans and place in a large covered pot. Add chicken broth and water and bring to a boil. Uncover pot, reduce heat, and simmer until beans are tender; roughly 1 hour. Add potatoes, pasta, carrots, celery, onion, garlic, and tomato juice. Return mixture to a boil, then reduce heat and simmer uncovered for 10 minutes. Add tomatoes and zucchini, and simmer until all are tender. Process pesto ingredients in a food processor or blender until finely chopped. Remove soup from heat and stir in pesto mixture, and serve garnished with Parmesan cheese if desired.

Approx. 182 calories per serving without pesto
10g protein, 1g total fat, 0 saturated fat, 0 trans fat,
20g carbohydrates, 3mg cholesterol, 204mg sodium, 4g fiber

Approx. 254 calories per serving with pesto added
12g protein, 8g total fat, 2g saturated fat, 0 trans fat,
20g carbohydrates, 10mg cholesterol, 291mg sodium, 4g fiber

CHILLY TOMATO SOUP
(MAKES 4 SERVINGS)

10 medium ripe tomatoes
½ tablespoon extra-virgin olive oil
1–5 cloves garlic, minced
2 tablespoons chopped onions
2 cups low-sodium, fat-free chicken broth
2 teaspoons low-calorie baking sweetener
½ teaspoon fresh basil, chopped

Salt and freshly ground pepper to taste
8 scallions, chopped (optional)
2 cucumbers, diced (optional)
1 large green zucchini, diced (optional)

In a large pot of boiling water, dip tomatoes for 30 seconds, then immediately place tomatoes in cold water. Allow to sit until they can be handled. Skin tomatoes with a paring knife, cut in half crosswise, and remove seeds. Core and then cut into quarter pieces. In a blender or food processor, process tomatoes until pureed. In a skillet, heat olive oil and sauté garlic and onions until tender. Remove from heat. In a large bowl, combine pureed tomatoes, sautéed onion mixture, chicken broth, sweetener, basil, and salt and pepper, stirring to mix ingredients together. Refrigerate soup for 4–6 hours until well chilled. Garnish with scallions, cucumbers, and zucchini if desired.

Approx. 161 calories per serving
10g protein, <0.5g total fat, 0 saturated fat, 0 trans fat,
65g carbohydrates, 5mg cholesterol, 197mg sodium, 1g fiber

HEARTY BEAN SOUP
(MAKES 6–8 SERVINGS)

2 cups water
2 medium potatoes, peeled and coarsely chopped
2 large carrots, coarsely chopped
2 stalks celery, coarsely chopped
1 bay leaf
1 tablespoon fresh thyme
Salt and freshly ground pepper to taste
3 tablespoons extra-virgin olive oil
5 cloves fresh garlic, minced
1 medium onion, finely chopped
½ small hot pepper, finely chopped
5 cups low-sodium, fat-free chicken broth
4 (15-ounce) cans Great Northern beans
Grated Parmesan cheese (optional)
Chopped fresh flat leaf parsley (optional)

In a heavy pot, combine water, potato, carrots, celery, bay leaf, thyme, and salt and pepper. Bring to a boil, reduce heat, cover, and simmer until vegetables are tender. While vegetables are cooking, combine oil, garlic, onion, and hot pepper in a large skillet, and sauté until tender and lightly browned. Add 1 cup of chicken broth and beans to garlic mixture, mix together well, cover, and simmer for about 10 minutes to allow flavors to blend. Add salt and pepper to taste. Combine bean mixture and 4 cups of chicken broth, and add to vegetable pot. Stir to mix, then keep at a low simmer for about 10–15 minutes, allowing flavors to blend. Garnish with cheese and parsley, if desired.

Approx. 220 calories per serving
11g protein, 6g total fat, 0.7g saturated fat, 0 trans fat,
36g carbohydrates, 3mg cholesterol, 663mg sodium, 9g fiber

EGGPLANT SOUP
(MAKES 4–6 SERVINGS)

2 tablespoons extra-virgin olive oil
2 cloves fresh garlic, minced
½ medium onion, thinly sliced and separated into rings
1 medium eggplant, peeled and cut into ½-inch cubes
½ teaspoon oregano
¼ teaspoon thyme
4 cups low-sodium, fat-free chicken broth
½ cup dry sherry
Salt and freshly ground pepper to taste
1 large tomato, sliced
10 ounces crumbled non-fat feta cheese
Freshly grated Parmesan cheese (optional)

Heat oil in large skillet over medium heat; add garlic and onion, and sauté until lightly golden. Add eggplant, oregano, and thyme; continue cooking until eggplant browns slightly, stirring constantly. Reduce heat to low, add broth, cover, and simmer for roughly 5 minutes. Add sherry, cover, and continue to simmer for another 2–3 minutes. Stir in salt and pepper to taste if needed, and remove from heat. Allow to cool slightly. Preheat broiler, and pour slightly cooled soup into an oven-safe bowl. Top soup with tomato slices and feta cheese, place soup under broiler, and heat until feta melts into soup. Garnish with grated Parmesan cheese if desired, and broil until cheese is browned.

Approx. 146 calories per serving
9g protein, 5g total fat, <1g saturated fat, 0 trans fat,
10g carbohydrates, 3mg cholesterol, 538mg sodium, 2g fiber

Pizza

PIZZA MARGHERITA
(MAKES AN 8-SLICE, 15-INCH PIZZA)

Thin Crust Pizza Dough (page 214)
4 Roma tomatoes, thinly sliced
Salt and freshly ground pepper to taste
½ cup yellow sweet pepper, thinly sliced
¾ cup shredded part-skim mozzarella cheese, about 3 ounces
4–5 snipped fresh basil leaves
¼ cup freshly grated Parmesan cheese
1 tablespoon extra-virgin olive oil

Preheat oven to 450 degrees. Follow directions for pizza dough and roll out to a 12–15-inch round. Place dough on a scantly oiled pizza pan. Spread tomatoes on rolled-out dough almost to the edge of the crust. Sprinkle with salt and pepper to taste. Top tomatoes with yellow peppers, mozzarella cheese, basil, and Parmesan cheese, and drizzle olive oil over the top. Bake at 450 degrees for 8–10 minutes or until crust is crisp and cheeses are melted.

Approx. 202 calories per slice
11g protein, 7g total fat, 3g saturated fat, 0 trans fat,
28g carbohydrates, 7mg cholesterol, 375mg sodium, 1g fiber

THIN CRUST PIZZA DOUGH
(MAKES AN 8-SLICE, 15-INCH CRUST)

1⅔ cups unbleached all-purpose flour
½ teaspoon salt
1 package dry active yeast
2 tablespoons extra-virgin olive oil
½ cup warm water
Olive oil to lightly coat pan

Put flour, salt, and yeast in a large bowl and mix with a wooden spoon. Make a well in the center and add oil and water. Gradually work in flour from the sides of the bowl as the mixture becomes smooth, pliable, soft dough. If too sticky, sprinkle a little more flour into the mixture, but don't make the dough dry. Transfer dough to a lightly floured surface and knead for about 10 minutes; add very small amounts of flour if needed until dough becomes smooth and elastic. Rub a small amount of oil over the surface of the dough, then return it to a clean bowl, cover it with a cloth, and place it in a warm area for about 1 hour or until dough doubles in size. Remove dough to a lightly floured surface, knead for an additional 2 minutes, then roll out into a 15-inch round. Place on pizza pan and top with sauce and ingredients of choice. Bake at 425 degrees until crust is crispy.

Approx. 115 calories per slice, crust only
2g protein, 3g total fat, <0.5g saturated fat, 0 trans fat,
18g carbohydrates, 0 cholesterol, 144mg sodium, 0 fiber

Wraps and Sandwiches

CHICKPEA PITA POCKETS
(MAKES 8 SERVINGS)

1 (15-ounce) can chickpeas, rinsed and drained
1 cup shredded fresh spinach
⅔ cup halved seedless red grapes
½ cup finely chopped red bell pepper

⅓ cup thinly sliced celery
½ medium cucumber, diced
¼ cup finely chopped onion
¼ cup light mayonnaise
1 tablespoon balsamic syrup
½ tablespoon poppy seed
4 (6-inch) whole wheat pita loaves, cut in half

In a large bowl combine chickpeas, spinach, grapes, red pepper, celery, cucumber, and onion. Whisk together mayonnaise, balsamic syrup, and poppy seeds. Add poppy seed mixture to chickpea mixture, and stir until well blended. Lightly toast pita halves and fill with chickpea filling. Serve.

Approx. 152 calories per serving
7g protein, 3g total fat, 0.3g saturated fat, 0 trans fat,
29g carbohydrates, 3mg cholesterol, 294mg sodium, 5g fiber

VEGGIE WRAP
(MAKES 6 SERVINGS)

Olive oil cooking spray
2 medium tomatoes, cut into ½-inch thick slices
2 small cucumbers, sliced lengthwise into ½-inch thick slices
2 small onions, cut into ½-inch thick slices
1 green bell pepper, cut into strips
2 medium zucchini, sliced lengthwise into ½-inch thick slices
Extra-virgin olive oil to drizzle
¾ tablespoon crumbled dried oregano
¼ tablespoon crumbled dried rosemary
¾ teaspoon dried thyme
½ (7-ounce) can chickpeas, rinsed and drained
¼ teaspoon cumin (optional)
Salt and freshly ground pepper to taste
6 whole wheat flat bread (8–10-inch), warmed
Alfalfa sprouts (optional)

Spray non-stick pan with cooking spray. Place tomatoes, cucumbers, onions, peppers, and zucchini on pan, and drizzle with olive oil. Sprinkle with oregano, rosemary, and thyme, and roast for 15–20 minutes at 425 degrees. Add chickpeas and cumin, plus salt and pepper to taste, and cook an additional 15–20 minutes until tender. Fill warmed flat bread with bean and veggie mix, top with alfalfa sprouts, roll up, and serve.

Approx. 170 calories per serving
8g protein, 1g total fat, <0.3g saturated fat, 0 trans fat,
36g carbohydrates, 0 cholesterol, 325mg sodium, 6g fiber

Main Dishes

LINGUINE AND MIXED SEAFOOD
(MAKES 4–6 SERVINGS)

8 ounces natural clam juice
2 cups good dry wine (not cooking wine)
¼ pound baby octopus, cleaned
¼ pound shrimp, peeled and deveined
¼ pound calamari, cleaned, cut into ¼-inch rings
20 mussels, scrubbed and debearded (discard any open mussels)
¼ pound bay scallops
3 tablespoons extra-virgin olive oil
3–4 cloves garlic, minced
¼ teaspoon freshly chopped hot peppers
8 small ripe plum tomatoes, chopped into small chunks
Pinch of low-calorie baking sweetener
½ tablespoon chopped fresh parsley
½ tablespoon chopped fresh oregano
Salt and freshly ground pepper to taste
½ pound linguine
10–12 arugula leaves, chopped
10 pitted Kalamata black olives, halved

In a large deep skillet, add clam juice, wine, octopus, shrimp, calamari, mussels, and scallops. Bring to boil, cover, and reduce heat to simmer, stirring occasionally, until calamari and squid are almost tender. Remove mussels and shell all but 9–12; set these aside for garnish and return shelled mussels to seafood skillet to keep warm. In a separate skillet, over medium heat, add oil and garlic, and sauté until golden brown. Add hot peppers to garlic mixture, reduce heat to simmer, and cook for 1–2 additional minutes. Add tomatoes, sweetener, parsley, oregano, and salt and pepper to taste, and simmer another 3–4 minutes. Cover to keep warm, and set aside. Bring water to a boil, add pasta, and cook pasta until *al dente*. Remove from heat, drain pasta, and return to pot, drizzling with scant amount of olive oil to keep pasta from sticking together. Set aside. With a slotted spoon remove seafood from skillet and strain remaining liquid through sieve or cheesecloth. Return seafood and 1 cup of strained liquid to skillet; add pasta and tomato mixture, and toss all ingredients. Spoon entire linguini and seafood dish into a large pasta bowl, garnish with chopped arugula, black olives, and remaining unshelled mussels, and serve.

Approx. 375 calories per serving
21g protein, 8g total fat, 1g saturated fat, 0 trans fat,
34g carbohydrates, 98mg cholesterol, 235mg sodium, 2g fiber

GRILLED CITRUS SALMON WITH GARLIC GREENS
(MAKES 4 SERVINGS)

¼ cup orange marmalade
2 tablespoons fresh lime juice
2 tablespoons fresh lemon juice
¼ cup low-sodium soy sauce
3 teaspoons grated orange rind
4 (3-ounce) salmon fillets
2 teaspoons extra-virgin olive oil
2 teaspoons minced garlic
2 (10-ounce) bags fresh spinach
Scant amount of olive oil to rub on fish
Salt and freshly ground pepper to taste
1 teaspoon fresh garlic, mashed to rub on fish
1 heaping tablespoon capers, drained
1 tablespoon balsamic vinegar
4 scallions, white and light green parts, thinly sliced (2–3-inch lengths)

Whisk together marmalade, lime and lemon juices, soy sauce, and orange rind; pour mixture over fillets and marinade for 30 minutes in refrigerator. Prepare grill or preheat broiler. Heat olive oil in a heavy skillet over medium-high heat; add garlic and spinach, one bag at a time, and sauté, stirring often, until spinach is wilted (about 2 minutes). Reduce heat to very low, to keep warm. Combine olive oil, salt and pepper, mashed garlic, and capers. Rub mixture into both sides of salmon steaks. Grill the fish or broil 3–4 inches from flame for 2–2 ½ minutes on each side. Set fish aside. Remove spinach from heat and toss with vinegar; divide equally on 4 plates. Add grilled salmon fillet to bed of spinach on each plate and garnish with onions. Serve.

Approx. 250 calories per serving
18g protein, 8g total fat, 1g saturated fat, 0 trans fat,
14g carbohydrates, 188mg cholesterol, 884mg sodium, 6g fiber

CHICKEN PICCATA
(MAKES 4 SERVINGS)

2 teaspoons extra-virgin olive oil
4 (3-ounce) skinless, boneless chicken breast fillets, lightly pounded
Salt and freshly ground pepper to taste
3 cloves fresh garlic, minced
1 cup low-sodium, fat-free chicken broth
2 tablespoon dry white wine
4 teaspoons lemon juice
1 tablespoon all-purpose flour
2 tablespoons chopped fresh parsley
1 tablespoon capers
Lemon wedges for garnish

Rinse chicken breast fillets under cold water and pat dry, then place breasts between layers of wax paper and lightly pound fillets with a meat mallet. Lightly sprinkle each fillet with salt and pepper if desired. Heat 1 teaspoon of olive oil in a large heavy-bottomed skillet over medium heat, add chicken fillets, and cook until fillets are lightly browned and centers cooked (juice will run clear). Transfer fillets to a serving platter and put in a low-temperature oven to keep warm. Add remaining teaspoon of oil and garlic to skillet and cook for 30 seconds to soften. Combine chicken broth, wine, lemon juice, and flour in skillet where chicken was cooked. Stir to blend, and continue stirring until mixture thickens. Add parsley and capers to sauce. Remove chicken from oven, place each fillet on a plate, and spoon mixture over fillets. Garnish with lemon wedges. Serve with cooked spinach linguine or pasta of choice.

Approx. 223 calories per serving
21g protein, 11g total fat, 2g saturated fat, 0 trans fat,
4g carbohydrates, 48mg cholesterol, 380mg sodium, <0.5g fiber

SPICY WHOLE WHEAT CAPELLINI WITH GARLIC
(MAKES 4 SERVINGS)

8 ounces whole wheat capellini pasta
¼ cup extra-virgin olive oil
4 cloves garlic, chopped
1 teaspoon diced hot peppers
Salt and freshly ground pepper to taste
Grated Pecorino or Parmesan cheese (optional)

Bring water to a boil, add pasta, and cook pasta until *al dente*. Remove from heat, drain pasta, and return to pot, drizzling with scant amount of olive oil to keep pasta from sticking together. Set aside. In a heavy skillet over medium heat, add olive oil, then sauté garlic and hot pepper until tender (about 1–2 minutes). Add to pasta and toss. Add salt and pepper to taste, and sprinkle with grated cheese if desired.

Approx. 299 calories per serving
8g protein, 16g total fat, 2g saturated fat, 0 trans fat,
35g carbohydrates, 4mg cholesterol, 0 sodium, 7g fiber

FETTUCCINE WITH SMOKED SALMON AND BASIL PESTO
(MAKES 4 SERVINGS)

8 ounces dried whole grain fettuccine pasta
Drizzle of extra-virgin olive oil
¼ cup Fresh Basil Pesto Sauce (Option: See page 357 of The Miami
Mediterranean Diet) *or market-fresh pesto*

10 pitted black olives, halved
½ tablespoon capers, rinsed well and drained
6 ounces nova smoked salmon (cut into thin strips)
1 tablespoon freshly grated Romano cheese
4 sprigs fresh basil leaves for garnish

Bring water to a boil, add pasta, and cook pasta until *al dente*. Remove from heat, drain pasta, and return to pot, drizzling with scant amount of olive oil to keep pasta from sticking together. Set aside. Meanwhile, warm pesto sauce in a saucepan under low heat, add olives and capers, remove from heat and add salmon. In a large serving bowl, toss pasta with salmon mixture. Divide into 4 portions, and serve with ¼ tablespoon of cheese, garnished with a fresh basil sprig.

Approx. 323 calories per serving
15g protein, 10g total fat, 2g saturated fat, 0 trans fat,
44g carbohydrates, 14mg cholesterol, 540mg sodium, <1g fiber

BAKED TILAPIA
(MAKES 2 SERVINGS)

4 (4-ounce) tilapia fillets
2 tablespoons extra-virgin olive oil
3 cloves garlic, minced
2 scallions, white and green parts, chopped
½ cup fresh chopped parsley
Salt and freshly ground pepper to taste
Fresh spinach leaves and 6 grape tomatoes, halved, for garnish
Juice from 2 lemons
1 lemon, quartered

Rinse fillets under cold water and pat dry. Place fillets in a baking dish. In mixing bowl combine oil, garlic, scallions, and parsley; pour over fish, cover, and refrigerate for 30 minutes. Sprinkle with salt and pepper and bake at 350 degrees for 15 minutes or until fish flakes easily. Divide cleaned spinach on 2 plates. Remove fish from oven, and place 2 fillets on top of spinach on each plate. Garnish each plate with tomato halves. Squeeze juice from 2 lemons over fillets, garnish with lemon wedge, and serve.

Approx. 138 calories per serving (two fillets per serving)
15g protein, 8g total fat, 1g saturated fat, 0 trans fat,
3g carbohydrates, 43mg cholesterol, 46mg sodium, 0 fiber

FETTUCCINE WITH SUNDRIED TOMATOES AND GOAT CHEESE
(MAKES 6–8 SERVINGS)

4 tablespoons chopped sundried tomatoes (in olive oil)
1 cup sliced scallions
4 garlic cloves, minced
1 medium red bell pepper, thinly sliced
½ cup dry vermouth
¼ cup chopped fresh basil
10 pitted Kalamata olives
1 tablespoon capers, rinsed and drained
2 teaspoons dried oregano
1 pound whole wheat fettuccine, cooked and drained
6 ounces low-fat goat cheese, crumbled

Drain oil from tomatoes and reserve oil; set tomatoes aside. In a large skillet, heat oil from tomatoes over medium heat. Add scallions and garlic to oil and sauté until soft. Add red peppers and ¼ cup of vermouth to garlic mixture. Cook peppers until crispy tender or until vermouth is almost evaporated. Reduce heat to simmer, and add tomatoes, remaining ¼ cup of vermouth, basil, olives, capers, and oregano. Simmer, stirring often to incorporate flavors (about 5–8 minutes), then reduce to very low heat to keep warm. Cook pasta to desired consistency (*al dente* would be best), and drain. Place pasta in a large bowl and toss with goat cheese until well blended. Add tomato mixture and toss again until well mixed. Serve.

Approx. 269 calories per serving
12g protein, 6g total fat, 2g saturated fat, 0 trans fat,
44g carbohydrates, 4mg cholesterol, 323mg sodium, 7g fiber

Side Dishes

GRILLED EGGPLANT
(MAKES 4 SERVINGS)

1 tablespoon extra-virgin olive oil
2 tablespoons fresh oregano leaves
2 plum tomatoes, diced
1½ pounds eggplant, cut lengthwise into ½-inch thick slices
Olive oil cooking spray
2 large garlic cloves, finely minced
1 teaspoon chopped dried rosemary
Salt and freshly ground pepper to taste
¼ cup crumbled feta cheese
Lemon wedges
Oregano sprigs for garnish

Heat oil in saucepan, add oregano leaves, then remove pan from heat. Add tomato to oregano and allow to bathe in hot oil until ready to serve. Meanwhile, spray both sides of eggplant with olive oil spray, sprinkle with garlic, rosemary, and salt and pepper, and place on medium-hot grill. Cover grill and cook eggplant until tender and browned on both sides, turning once. Remove eggplant to platter, drizzle with oregano tomato oil, and top with feta cheese. Garnish with lemon wedges and oregano sprigs.

Approx. 74 calories per serving
4g protein, 6g total fat, 1g saturated fat, 0 trans fat,
10g carbohydrates, 5mg cholesterol, 86mg sodium, 0.2g fiber

ROASTED PEPPERS
(MAKES 4–6 SERVINGS)

4 large red bell peppers
2 cloves garlic, peeled and sliced
4 tablespoons extra-virgin olive oil
Salt and freshly ground pepper to taste

Clean peppers and pat dry. Place peppers on moderately hot grill or on a rack under a broiler 1–2 inches from heat, turning often until skin is charred and blistered. Charring of entire skin takes about 15–20 minutes. Remove from grill or broiler and place peppers aside to cool. When cool enough to handle, rub off blackened skins. Cut each pepper in half, remove stalk and seeds, and cut into ½-inch strips. Place strips in a bowl, and add garlic, oil, and salt and pepper to taste. Toss and set aside for about 30 minutes before serving.

Approx. 108 calories per serving
1g protein, 10g total fat, 1g saturated fat, 0 trans fat,
7g carbohydrates, 0 cholesterol, 2mg sodium, 2g fiber

CLASSIC SPINACH AND PINE NUTS
(MAKES 4 SERVINGS)

¼ cup golden raisins
4 tablespoons pine nuts
2 tablespoons extra-virgin olive oil
4 cloves garlic, chopped
1½ (10-ounce) bags fresh spinach, cleaned
Fresh lemon juice
Extra-virgin olive oil to taste
Salt and freshly ground pepper to taste

Place raisins in a bowl and cover with boiling water. Let stand for approximately 10 minutes, until raisins are plump; drain well. In a skillet over medium heat, toast pine nuts, stirring constantly for about 1–2 minutes. Remove from heat, and set aside. In a large skillet, warm olive oil. Add garlic and sauté for 1–2 minutes, until golden. Add spinach a little at a time until it all becomes wilted (about 3–5 minutes), stirring constantly. Pour raisins over spinach and mix well. With a slotted spoon, transfer spinach to a serving dish, and sprinkle pine nuts over top. Serve immediately or, if serving at room temperature, add fresh lemon juice and extra-virgin olive oil and salt and pepper to taste.

Approx. 149 calories per serving
4g protein, 12g total fat, 2g saturated fat, 0 trans fat,
10g carbohydrates, 0 cholesterol, 41mg sodium, 2g fiber

BROCCOLI WITH FRESH GARLIC
(MAKES 4–6 SERVINGS)

10–12 fresh broccoli spears, roughly 6 inches long
3 cups low-sodium, fat-free chicken broth
3 tablespoons extra-virgin olive oil
2–3 cloves fresh garlic, crushed
2 tablespoons chopped fresh parsley
Salt to taste
Pinch of freshly ground pepper to taste

Cook spears in a large skillet of chicken broth until slightly under-cooked (about 7 minutes). Test with a fork; do not overcook. Drain well and set aside. Heat oil in a large skillet over medium-high heat; add garlic and sauté until golden brown. Add broccoli, parsley, and seasonings to taste. Turn broccoli several times, mixing well with seasonings, oil, and garlic. Serve immediately.

Approx. 161 calories per serving
11g protein, 9g total fat, 2g saturated fat, 0 trans fat,
16g carbohydrates, 1mg cholesterol, 80mg sodium, 9g fiber

Desserts

DRUNKEN APRICOTS
(MAKES 4 SERVINGS)

8 medium apricots
1½ cups red wine
1⅓ cups water
3 strips lemon peel (yellow part only)
3 tablespoons honey
1 cinnamon stick
Sprinkle with non-caloric sweetener to taste (optional)
Fat-free whipped cream (optional)

Peel skin from apricots. In a saucepan add wine, water, lemon peel, honey, and cinnamon stick, and bring to boil. Add apricots to sauce, submerging under liquid as much as possible, and gently poach for 5–10 minutes, until just tender. Remove apricots from saucepan and place in a bowl; set aside. Boil liquid in the saucepan, stirring constantly, until it becomes thick and syrupy. Remove cinnamon stick and lemon peel before liquid becomes dark. Pour syrup, when cool, over apricots, and serve. Garnish with sweetener and whipped cream if desired.

Approx. 112 calories per serving
1g protein, 0.3g total fat, 0 saturated fat, 0 trans fat,
20g carbohydrates, 0 cholesterol, 1mg sodium, 1g fiber

STRAWBERRIES AND BALSAMIC SYRUP
(MAKES 4 SERVINGS)

2½ cups strawberries, hulled and halved
4 tablespoons Crème de Banana liqueur
Non-caloric sweetener to taste
Balsamic syrup

Combine strawberries and liqueur in a large bowl, toss well, cover, and refrigerate 20–30 minutes. When ready to serve, remove strawberries with a slotted spoon and place in a single layer on a dessert platter. Dust generously with sweetener, drizzle with balsamic syrup, and serve.

Approx. 49 calories per serving
<1g protein, 0.4g total fat, <0.1g saturated fat, 0 trans fat,
7g carbohydrates, 0 cholesterol, 1mg sodium, 2g fiber

HONEYDEW SORBET
(MAKES 4–6 SERVINGS)

1½ cups of water
½ cup low-calorie baking sweetener
2 ripe honeydews (about 5 inches in diameter each), peeled, seeded,
    and chunked
¼ cup fresh lemon juice
¼ cup egg whites
Mint sprigs for garnish

Combine water and sweetener, and bring to a boil over medium heat. Reduce heat and simmer for 5 minutes, then allow to cool. In a food processor or blender add honeydew and its juices, lemon juice, and cooled syrup. Puree until smooth. Pour mixture into bowl and freeze until almost frozen. Remove from freezer and beat with an electric beater until mixture is again smooth. Beat egg white until stiff and fold into frozen fruit mixture. Cover container and freeze again until firm (about 2–3 hours). When ready to serve, scoop into dessert cups and garnish with mint sprigs if desired.

Approx. 117 calories per serving
2g protein, <0.5g total fat, 0 saturated fat, 0 trans fat,
31g carbohydrates, 0 cholesterol, 33mg sodium, 2g fiber

MERINGUE COOKIES
(MAKES 20–24 COOKIES)

1 cup liquid egg whites
Pinch of cream of tartar
¼ cup low-calorie baking sweetener
1 teaspoon white wine vinegar
1 teaspoon vanilla extract

Line 2 cookie trays with parchment paper. Place egg whites in a mixing bowl and slowly whisk on low speed with an electric beater until they begin to bubble. Add cream of tartar and increase speed slightly; whisk until the mixture begins to peak. Increase speed to medium and slowly add sweetener, vinegar, and vanilla extract. Continue whisking until mixture is satiny and firmly holds peak. Ladle a soup spoon-sized portion of mixture onto parchment-lined trays to make 20–24 cookies. Put trays of meringues in an oven preheated to 275 degrees to bake for about 1 hour. Turn off oven and allow cookies to stand in closed oven for an additional hour to dry. When meringues are pierced with a toothpick that comes back dry, they are ready. Transfer cookies to cooling racks to continue to cool.

Approx. 5 calories per cookie
1g protein, 0 total fat, 0 saturated fat, 0 trans fat,
<0.1g carbohydrates, 0 cholesterol, 15mg sodium, 0 fiber

SWEET PLUM COMPOTE
(MAKES 6 SERVINGS)

Canola oil cooking spray
3 pounds ripe plums, halved and pitted
¼ cup low-calorie baking sweetener
1 cup water
1 tablespoon Crème de Cassis liqueur

Lightly spray a baking dish with cooking spray. Add plums to baking dish. Combine sweetener and water in a saucepan and bring to a boil; cook for about 5 minutes, stirring constantly, or until liquid becomes syrupy. Pour syrup over plums and drizzle with Crème de Cassis. Bake mixture for 45 minutes to 1 hour in a 350-degree oven. Serve warm or cool.

Approx. 130 calories per serving
2g protein, 1g total fat, 0.1g saturated fat, 0 trans fat,
28g carbohydrates, 0 cholesterol, 1mg sodium, 1g fiber

PEACH MARSALA COMPOTE
(MAKES 6 SERVINGS)

Canola oil cooking spray
12 fresh peaches
6 cups water
¾ cup low-calorie baking sweetener
½ cup Marsala wine
½ teaspoon ground cinnamon
½ teaspoon vanilla extract
½ teaspoon freshly grated nutmeg

Lightly spray a 2-quart baking dish with cooking spray. Blanch the peaches in boiling water for 20 seconds, then remove skin while holding under cold running water. Pit and slice peaches. Add peaches, sweetener, wine, cinnamon, vanilla extract, and nutmeg to a baking dish and bake for 45 minutes to 1 hour in a 350-degree oven. Serve warm or at room temperature.

Approx. 80 calories per serving
1g protein, 0.2g total fat, 0 saturated fat, 0 trans fat,
21g carbohydrates, 0 cholesterol, 126mg sodium, 3g fiber

STRAWBERRIES AMARETTO
(MAKES 8 SERVINGS)

3 pints fresh strawberries
2 cups plain low-fat yogurt
1 teaspoon vanilla extract
¼ cup Amaretto liqueur
Fat-free whipped cream (if desired)

Set aside 8 strawberries for garnish. Hull remaining strawberries and cut into halves. Place strawberry halves in dessert cups. In a bowl combine yogurt, vanilla extract, and liqueur; blend well. Pour over strawberries and garnish each cup with a reserved berry. Add whipped cream if desired.

Approx. 96 calories per serving
4g protein, 0.6g total fat, <0.5 saturated fat, 0 trans fat,
9g carbohydrates, <0.5mg cholesterol, 42mg sodium, 3g fiber

FRESH FRUIT KABOBS AND CINNAMON HONEY DIP
(MAKES 2 SERVINGS)

Assorted bite-sized chunks of your favorite fresh fruits (enough for 2
*   [8-inch] wooden skewers)*
1 cup of low-fat plain yogurt
2 tablespoons of honey or non-caloric sweetener
Pinch of ground white pepper
6 teaspoons of ground cinnamon or to taste

Prepare fruits on skewers and set aside. Combine yogurt, honey, and white pepper, and mix well. Divide mixture into two individual serving bowls; sprinkle cinnamon on top of each serving and gently swirl in. Cover and refrigerate to chill before serving.

NOTE: Values shown are for yogurt dip only (values for fruit cannot be calculated since they depend on the specific fruits chosen).

Approx. 70 calories per serving
0.5g protein, 2g total fat, 1g saturated fat, 0 trans fat,
8g carbohydrates, 7mg cholesterol, 75mg sodium, 0 fiber

Bibliography
and Further Reading

Part I: The Problem

Chapter 1: The Heart Surgery Hoax

Adler, Robert E. *Medical Firsts: From Hippocrates to the Human Genome.* Hoboken, NJ: Wiley, 2004.

Griffin, K. "No more knife guys." *AARP Magazine,* Nov.–Dec. 2004.

Kannel, W. B. "Clinical misconceptions dispelled by epidemiological research." *Circulation* 92 (1995): 3350–360.

Keys, A., A. Menotti, et al. "The seven countries study: 2,289 deaths in 15 years." *Preventative Medicine* 13 (1984): 141–54.

Keys, A. "Mediterranean diet and public health: personal reflections." *American Journal of Clinical Nutrition* 61 (1995): 1321S–323S.

Kolata, G. "The Limits of Opening Arteries." *New York Times,* 28 Mar. 2004.

Loudon, Irvine, ed. *Western Medicine: An Illustrated History.* Oxford: Oxford UP, 1997.

Mancini, M., and J. Stamler. "Diet for preventing cardiovascular diseases: light from Ancel Keys, distinguished centenarian scientist." *Nutrition, Metabolism & Cardiovascular Diseases* 14 (2004): 52–57.

Menotti, A., and A. Keys. "Seven Countries Study. First 20-year mortality data in 12 cohorts of six countries." *Annals of Internal Medicine* 21 (1989): 175–79.

Pitsavos, C., D. B. Panagiotakos, et al. "Forty-year follow-up of coronary heart disease mortality and its predictors: the Corfu cohort of the seven countries study." *Preventative Cardiology* 6 (2003): 155–60.

Trichopoulou, A. "Mediterranean diet: the past and the present." *Nutrition, Metabolism & Cardiovascular Diseases* 11 (2001): 1–4.

Chapter 2: Heart Disease—It's Not Worth Dying For!

Fauci, Anthony S., Eugene Braunwald, Dennis L. Kasper, and Stephan L. Hauser. *Harrison's Principles of Internal Medicine V1.* New York: McGraw-Hill Companies, The, 2008.

Libby, Peter, P. M. Ridker, and A. Maseri. "Inflammation and atherosclerosis." *Circulation* 105 (2002): 1135–143.

Libby, Peter, Robert O. Bonow, Douglas L. Mann, and Douglas P. Zipes, eds. *Braunwald's Heart Disease: A Textbook of Cardiovascular Medicine.* Philadelphia: Saunders, 2007.

Murphy, Joseph G., ed. *Mayo Clinic Cardiology Review.* New York: Informa Healthcare, 2006.

Walsh, Richard A., Philip Poole-Wilson, and Spencer B. King, eds. *Hurst's the Heart.* New York: McGraw-Hill Professional, 2007.

Chapter 3: Understanding Heart Surgery

Alderman, E. L., and M. G. Bourassa. "Ten-year follow-up of survival and myocardial infarction in the randomized Coronary Artery Surgery Study." *Circulation* 82 (1990): 1629–646.

Captur, G. "Memento for René Favaloro." *Texas Heart Institute Journal* 31 (2004): 47–60.

Caracciolo, E. A., K. B. Davis, et al. "Comparison of surgical and medical group survival in patients with left main equivalent coronary artery disease. Long-term CASS experience." *Circulation* 91 (1995): 2335–344.

Chaitman, B. R., T. J. Ryan, et al. "Coronary Artery Surgery Study (CASS): comparability of 10 year survival in randomized and randomizable patients." *Journal of the American College of Cardiology* 16 (1990): 1071–078.

"Eighteen-year follow-up in the Veterans Affairs Cooperative Study of Coronary Artery Bypass Surgery for stable angina. The VA Coronary Artery Bypass Surgery Cooperative Study Group." *Circulation* 86 (1992): 121–30.

"Eleven-year survival in the Veterans Administration randomized trial of coronary bypass surgery for stable angina. The Veterans Administration Coronary Artery Bypass Surgery Cooperative Study Group." *New England Journal of Medicine* 311 (1984): 1333–339.

Libby, Peter, Robert O. Bonow, Douglas L. Mann, and Douglas P. Zipes, eds. *Braunwald's Heart Disease: A Textbook of Cardiovascular Medicine.* Philadelphia: Saunders, 2007.

Myers, W. O., E. H. Blackstone, et al. "CASS Registry long term surgical survival. Coronary Artery Surgery Study." *Journal of the American College of Cardiology* 33 (1999): 488–98.

Myers, W. O., K. Davis, et al. "Surgical survival in the Coronary Artery Surgery Study (CASS) registry." *Annals of Thoracic Surgery* 40 (1985): 245–60.

Peduzzi, P., A. Kamina, and K. Detre. "Twenty-two-year follow-up in the VA Cooperative Study of Coronary Artery Bypass Surgery for Stable Angina." *American Journal of Cardiology* 81 (1998): 1393–399.

Chapter 4: Why Bypass Surgery and Angioplasty Seldom Work and Why We Keep Doing Them Anyway

Griffin, K. "No more knife guys." *AARP Magazine,* Nov.–Dec. 2004.

Hochman, J. S., and G. A. Lamas. "Coronary intervention for persistent occlusion after myocardial infarction." *New England Journal of Medicine* 355 (2006): 2395–407.

Hueb, W. A., and P. R. Soares. "Five-year follow-up of the medicine, angioplasty, or surgery study (MASS): A prospective, randomized trial of medical therapy, balloon angioplasty, or bypass surgery for single proximal left anterior descending coronary artery stenosis." *Circulation* 100 (1999): II107–I113.

Katritsis, D. G., and J. P. Ioannidis. "Percutaneous coronary intervention versus conservative therapy in nonacute coronary artery disease: a meta-analysis." *Circulation* 111 (2005): 2906–912.

Kolata, G. "The Limits of Opening Arteries." *New York Times,* 28 Mar. 2004.

Ornish, Dean. *Dr. Dean Ornish's Program for Reversing Heart Disease.* New York: Ivy Books, 1997.

Update to FDA Statement on Coronary Drug-Eluting Stents. Department of Health and Human Services. U.S. Food and Drug Administration. 4 Jan. 2007. Center for Devices and Radiological Health. 11 Feb. 2008 <http://www.fda.gov/cdrh/news/010407.html>.

Whitaker, Julian M. *Reversing Heart Disease: A Vital New Program to Help, Treat, and Eliminate Cardiac Problems Without Surgery.* Grand Rapids: Grand Central, 2002.

Chapter 5: Pharmaceutical Follies

Abramson, John. *Overdosed America: The Broken Promise of American Medicine.* New York: HarperCollins, 2004.

Angell, Marcia. *The Truth about the Drug Companies: How They Deceive Us and What to Do about It.* New York: Random House, 2004.

Chapter 6: The Radiation Ruse

"64-Slice CT Scan." *Oregon Health & Science University.* 7 Nov. 2007 <http://www.ohsu.edu/health/page.cfm?id=13475>.

Brenner, D. J., and E. J. Hall. "Computed tomography—an increasing source of radiation exposure." *New England Journal of Medicine* 357 (2007): 2277–284.

"Body Scans. Do you know the risk?" *Life Extension,* Nov. 2001.

Brody, J. E. "Personal health; how perils can await the worried wealthy." *New York Times,* 12 Nov. 2002.

Cheng, T. O. "Siesta and coronary artery disease." *International Journal of Epidemiology* 30 (2001):183–4.

Clark, C. "Latest scanning device finds heart disease, and controversy, quickly." *San Diego Union-Tribune,* 1 Oct. 2006.

Coles, D. R., M. A. Smail, and I. S. Negus. "Comparison of radiation doses from multislice computed tomography coronary angiography and conventional diagnostic angiography." *Journal of the American College of Cardiology* 47 (2006): 1840–845.

"Computed Tomography Imaging (CT Scan, CAT Scan)." *Imaginis.* 13 Sept. 2007. 11 Dec. 2007 <http://www.imaginis.com/ct-scan/history.asp>.

Department of Environment and Climate Change. 3 Jan. 2008 <http://www.epa.nsw.gov.au/resources/ctbodyscan.pdf>.

Frush, Donald. "Cancer Risk From CAT Scans: Why You Shouldn't Worry." *ABC News.* 6 Nov. 2007.

Gorman, C. "How new heart-scanning technology could save your life" *Time*, 28 Aug. 2005.

Grady, D. "In a former first family, cancer has a grim legacy." *New York Times*, 7 Aug. 2007.

Harman, D. "Free radical theory of aging: an update: increasing the functional life span." *Annals of the New York Academy of Science*. 1067 (2006):10–21.

Harman, D. "Free radical theory of aging." *Mutation Research*. 275(1992): 257–66.

"Information on whole body scanning." New South Wales Government Department of Environment and Climate Change. 3 Dec. 2008 <http://www.environment.nsw.gov.au/radiation/ct-bodyscans.htm>.

Kalayoglu, Murat V. "64-slice CT and the New Age for Cardiac Diagnostics." *Medcompare*. 7 Nov. 2007 <http://www.medcompare.com/spotlight.asp?spotlightid=147>.

Masters, C. "Should you have a CT scan?" *Time*, 17 July 2007.

Mollet, N. R., F. Cademartiri, C. A. Van Mieghem, et al. "High-resolution spiral computed tomography coronary angiography in patients referred for diagnostic conventional coronary angiography." *Circulation* 112 (2005): 2318–323.

Ozner, M. "Avoiding the Radiation Dangers of Cardiac CAT Scans": *Life Extension Magazine*. March 2008.

Rabin, R. C. "The consumer: with rise in radiation exposure, experts urge caution on tests." *New York Times*, 19 June 2007.

Redberg, R. F. "Computed tomographic angiography: more than just a pretty picture?" *Journal of the American College of Cardiology* 49 (2007): 1827–829.

"The Radiation Risk of CT Scanning." *Trusted.MD*. 2 May 2007. 27 Dec. 2007 <http://trusted.md/feed/items/system/2007/05/02/the_radiation_risk_of_ct_scanning>.

Waugh, N, C. Black, et al. "The effectiveness and cost-effectiveness of computed tomography screening for coronary artery disease: systematic review." *Health Technology Assessment*. 10 (2006): iii–iv, ix–x, 1–41.

"Whole Body Scanning: What are the Radiation Risks from CT?" U.S. Food and Drug Administration. 27 Dec. 2007 <http://www.fda.gov/cdrh/ct/risks.html>.

Zaregarizi M, B. Edwards, et al. "Acute changes in cardiovascular function during the onset period of daytime sleep: comparison to lying awake and standing." *Journal of Applied Physiology.* 103 (2007): 1332–8.

Part II: The Solution

Step 1: Follow a Mediterranean Diet

Allen, J. P., M. Nelson, A. Alling. "The legacy of Biosphere 2 for the study of biospherics and closed ecological systems." *Advances in Space Research* 31 (2003): 1629–39.

Aronne, L. J., K. K. Isoldi. "Overweight and obesity: Key components of cardiometabolic risk." *Clinical Cornerstone* 8 (2007): 29–37.

Balk, E. M., A. H. Lichtenstein, et al. "Effects of omega-3 fatty acids on serum markers of cardiovascular disease risk: a systematic review." *Atherosclerosis* 189 (2006): 19–30.

Berger, J. S., D. L. Brown, R. C. Becker. "Low-dose aspirin in patients with stable cardiovascular disease: a meta-analysis." *American Journal of Medicine* 121 (2008): 43–9.

Bibbins-Domingo, K., P. Coxson, "Adolescent overweight and future adult coronary heart disease." *New England Journal of Medicine* 357 (2007): 2371–9.

Bray, G. A., S. J. Nielsen, B. M. Popkin. "Consumption of high-fructose corn syrup in beverages may play a role in the epidemic of obesity." *American Journal of Clinical Nutrition* 79 (2004): 537–43.

Brown, L., B. Rosner, et al. "Cholesterol-lowering effects of dietary fiber: a meta-analysis." *American Journal of Clinical Nutrition.*

Bruckert, E. "Abdominal obesity: A health threat." *Presse Med* (2008).

Burke, B. E., R. Neuenschwander, R. D. Olson. "Randomized, double-blind, placebo-controlled trial of coenzyme Q10 in isolated systolic hypertension." *Southern Medical Journal* 94 (2001): 1112–7.

Colomer, R., R. Lupu, et al. "Giacomo Castelvetro's salads. Anti-HER2 oncogene nutraceuticals since the 17th century?" *Clinical Translation Oncology* 10 (2008): 30–4.

Dannenberg, A. L., D. C. Burton, R. J. Jackson. "Economic and environmental costs of obesity: the impact on airlines." *American Journal of Preventive Medicine* 27 (2004): 264.

Djoussé, L, J. M. Gaziano. "Alcohol consumption and risk of heart failure in the Physicians' Health Study I." *Circulation* 115 (2007): 34–9.

Egan J. M., R. F. Margolskee. "Taste cells of the gut and gastrointestinal chemosensation." *Molecular Interventions* 8 (2008): 78–81.

Ellis, E. M. "Reactive carbonyls and oxidative stress: potential for therapeutic intervention." *Pharmacology & Therapeutics* 115 (2007): 13–24.

Ello-Martin, J. A., J. H. Ledikwe, B. J. Rolls. "The influence of food portion size and energy density on energy intake: implications for weight management." *American Journal of Clinical Nutrition* 82 (2005): 236S–241S.

Engler, M. M., M. B. Engler. "Omega-3 fatty acids: role in cardiovascular health and disease." *Journal of Cardiovascular Nursing* 21 (2006): 17–24, quiz 25–6.

Fontana, L. "Calorie restriction and cardiometabolic health." *European Journal of Cardiovascular Prevention and Rehabilitation* 15 (2008): 3–9.

Fontana, L. "Nutrition, adiposity and health." *Epidemiology Prevention* 31 (2007): 290–4.

Folts J. D. "The history of aspirin." *Texas Heart Institute Journal* 34 (2007): 392.

Forshee, R. A., M. L. Storey, et al. "A critical examination of the evidence relating high fructose corn syrup and weight gain." *Critical Reviews in Food Science and Nutrition* 47 (2007): 561–82.

Gaby, A. R. "Adverse effects of dietary fructose." *Alternative Medicine Review* 10 (2005): 294–306.

Harris, W. S. "Omega-3 fatty acids and cardiovascular disease: a case for omega-3 index as a new risk factor." *Pharmacology Research* 55 (2007): 217–23.

Holick, M. F., T. C. Chen. "Vitamin D deficiency: a worldwide problem with health consequences." *American Journal of Clinical Nutrition* 87 (2008): 1080S–6S.

Houston, M. C. "Treatment of hypertension with nutraceuticals, vitamins, antioxidants and minerals." *Expert Review of Cardiovascular Therapy* 5 (2007): 681–91.

Jacobs, D. R. Jr, L. F. Andersen, R. Blomhoff. "Whole-grain consumption is associated with a reduced risk of noncardiovascular, noncancer death attributed to inflammatory diseases in the Iowa Women's Health Study." *American Journal of Clinical Nutritition* 85 (2007): 1606–14.

Janson, M. "Orthomolecular medicine: the therapeutic use of dietary supplements for anti-aging." *Clinical Intervention in Aging* 1 (2006): 261–5.

Keys, A. "Mediterranean diet and public health: personal reflections." *American Journal of Clinical Nutrition* 61 (1995): 1321S–1323S.

Knoops, K.T., L. C. de Groot, et al. "Mediterranean diet, lifestyle factors, and 10-year mortality in elderly European men and women: the HALE project." *Journal of the American Medical Association* 292 (2004): 1433–9.

Konukoglu, D., G. D. Kemerli. "Protein carbonyl content in erythrocyte membranes in type 2 diabetic patients." *Hormone and Metabolic Research* 34 (2002): 367–70.

Lin, B. H., J. Guthrie, and E. Frazao. "Nutrient contribution of food away from home." *Agriculture Information Bulletin* No. 750. US Department of Agriculture. Economic Research Service. Ed. E. Frazao. Washington, DC, 1999. 213–39.

Malik, V. S., M. B. Schulze, F. B. Hu. "Intake of sugar-sweetened beverages and weight gain: a systematic review." *American Journal of Clinical Nutrition* 84 (2006): 274–88.

Mancini, M., and J. Stamler. "Diet for preventing cardiovascular diseases: light from Ancel Keys, distinguished centenarian scientist." *Nutrition, Metabolism & Cardiovascular Disease* 14 (2004): 52–7.

Maraldi, C., S. Volpato, et al. "Impact of inflammation on the relationship among alcohol consumption, mortality, and cardiac events: the health, aging, and body composition study." *Archives of Internal Medicine* 166 (2006): 1490–7.

Martini, L. A., R. J. Wood. "Vitamin D and blood pressure connection: update on epidemiologic, clinical, and mechanistic evidence." *Nutrition Review* 66 (2008): 291–7.

Maser, R. E., M. J. Lenhard. "An overview of the effect of weight loss on cardiovascular autonomic function." *Current Diabetes Review* 3 (2007): 204–11.

Miner, J., A. Hoffhines. "The discovery of aspirin's antithrombotic effects." *Texas Heart Institute Journal* 34 (2007): 179–86.

Mitrou, P. N., V. Kıpnıs, et al. "Mediterranean dietary pattern and prediction of all-cause mortality in a US population: results from the NIH-AARP Diet and Health Study." *Archives of Internal Medicine* 167 (2007): 2461–8.

Morrill, A. C., C. D. Chinn. "The obesity epidemic in the United States." *Journal of Public Health Policy* 25 (2004): 353–66.

Mozaffarian, D. "Trans fatty acids—effects on systemic inflammation and endothelial function." *Atherosclerosis Supplements* 7 (2006): 29–32.

Nakanishi, Y., K. Tsuneyama, et al. "Monosodium glutamate (MSG): a villain and promoter of liver inflammation and dysplasia." *Journal of Autoimmunity* 30 (2008): 42–50.

Odetti, P., S. Garibaldi, et al. "Levels of carbonyl groups in plasma proteins of type 2 diabetes mellitus subjects." *Acta Diabetologica* 36 (1999): 179–83.

O'Keefe, J. H., N. M. Gheewala, J. O. O'Keefe. "Dietary strategies for improving post-prandial glucose, lipids, inflammation, and cardiovascular health." *Journal of the American College of Cardiology* 51 (2008): 249–55.

Ozner, Michael. *The Miami Mediterranean Diet*. Dallas: BenBella Books, 2008.

Pennathur, S., J. W. Heinecke. "Mechanisms for oxidative stress in diabetic cardiovascular disease." *Antioxidants and Redox Signal* 9 (2007): 955–69.

Pennathur, S., Y. Ido, et al. "Reactive carbonyls and polyunsaturated fatty acids produce a hydroxyl radical-like species: a potential pathway for oxidative damage of retinal proteins in diabetes." *Journal of Biological Chemistry* 280 (2005): 22706–14.

Pergams, O. R., P. A. Zaradic. "Evidence for a fundamental and pervasive shift away from nature-based recreation." *Proceedings of the National Academy of Sciences (US)* (2008).

Pitsavos, C., D. B. Panagiotakos, et al. "Forty-year follow-up of coronary heart disease mortality and its predictors: the Corfu cohort of the seven countries study." *Preventative Cardiology* 6 (2003): 155–60.

Pradhan, A. "Obesity, metabolic syndrome, and type 2 diabetes: inflammatory basis of glucose metabolic disorders." *Nutrition Reviews* 65 (2007): S152–6.

Reaven, G., F. Abbasi, T. McLaughlin. "Obesity, insulin resistance, and cardiovascular disease." *Recent Progress in Hormone Research* 59 (2004): 207–23.

Schwalfenberg, G. "Omega-3 fatty acids: their beneficial role in cardiovascular health." *Canadian Family Physician* 52 (2006): 734–40.

Soriano-Guillen L, Hernandez-Garcia B, et al. "High Sensitivity C Reactive Protein Is a Good Marker of Cardiovascular Risk Factor in Obese Children and Adolescents." *European Journal of Endocrinology* (2008).

Tapsell, L. C., I. Hemphill, et al. "Health benefits of herbs and spices: the past, the present, the future." *Medical Journal of Australia* 185 (2006): S4–24.

Teff, K. L., S. S. Elliott, et al. "Dietary fructose reduces circulating insulin and leptin, attenuates postprandial suppression of ghrelin, and increases triglycerides in women." *Journal of Clinical Endocrinology and Metabolism* 89 (2004): 2963–72.

Tiano, L., R. Belardinelli, et al. "Effect of coenzyme Q10 administration on endothelial function and extracellular superoxide dismutase in patients with ischaemic heart disease: a double-blind, randomized controlled study." *European Heart Journal* 28 (2007): 2249–55.

Trichopoulou, A. "Mediterranean diet: the past and the present." *Nutrition, Metabolism & Cardiovascular Disease* 11 (2001): 1–4.

Vieth, R., H. Bischoff-Ferrari, et al. "The urgent need to recommend an intake of vitamin D that is effective." *American Journal of Clinical Nutrition* 85 (2007): 649–50.

Walford, R. L., D. Mock, et al. "Calorie restriction in biosphere 2: alterations in physiologic, hematologic, hormonal, and biochemical parameters in humans restricted for a 2-year period." *Journal of Gerontology Series A: Biological Sciences and Medical Sciences* 57 (2002): B211–24.

Wang, T. J., M. J. Pencina, et al. "Vitamin D deficiency and risk of cardiovascular disease." *Circulation* 117 (2008): 503–11.

Waterman, E, B. Lockwood. "Active components and clinical applications of olive oil." *Alternative Medicine Review* 12 (2007): 331–42.

Step 2: Exercise Regularly

Hamburg, N. M., C. J. McMackin, et al. "Physical inactivity rapidly induces insulin resistance and microvascular dysfunction in healthy volunteers." *Arteriosclerosis, Thrombosis, and Vascular Biology* 27 (2007): 2650–6.

Hewitt, J. A., G. P. Whyte, et al. "The effects of a graduated aerobic exercise programme on cardiovascular disease risk factors in the NHS workplace: a randomised controlled trial." *Journal of Occupational Medicine and Toxicology* (2008): 7.

Kruger, J., H. M. Blanck, C. Gillespie. "Dietary and physical activity behaviors among adults successful at weight loss maintenance." *International Journal of Behavioral Nutrition and Physical Activity* 3 (2006): 17.

Libby, Peter, Robert O. Bonow, Douglas L. Mann, and Douglas P. Zipes, eds. *Braunwald's Heart Disease: A Textbook of Cardiovascular Medicine*. Philadelphia: Saunders, 2007.

Puetz, T. W., S. S. Flowers, P. J. O'Connor. "A Randomized Controlled Trial of the Effect of Aerobic Exercise Training on Feelings of Energy and Fatigue in Sedentary Young Adults with Persistent Fatigue." *Psychotherapy and Psychosomatics* 77 (2008): 167–174.

Rendi, M., A. Szabo, et al. "Acute psychological benefits of aerobic exercise: A field study into the effects of exercise characteristics." *Psychology, Health & Medicine* 13 (2008): 180–4.

Schjerve, I. E., G. A. Tyldum, et al. "Both aerobic endurance and strength training programs improve cardiovascular health in obese adults." *Clinical Science* (2008).

Step 3: Manage Your Stress

Arthur, H. M., C. Patterson, J. A. Stone. "The role of complementary and alternative therapies in cardiac rehabilitation: a systematic evaluation." *European Journal of Cardiovascular Prevention & Rehabilitation* 13 (2006): 3–9.

Bennett, M. P., C. Lengacher. "Humor and Laughter May Influence Health: III. Laughter and Health Outcomes." *Evidence-based Complementary and Alternative Medicine* 5 (2008): 37–40.

Das, S., J. H. O'Keefe. "Behavioral cardiology: recognizing and addressing the profound impact of psychosocial stress on cardiovascular health." *Current Atherosclerosis Report* 8 (2006): 111–8.

Friedberg, J. P., S. Suchday, D. V. Shelov. "The impact of forgiveness on cardiovascular reactivity and recovery." *International Journal of Psycholphysiology* 65 (2007): 87–94.

Katzer, L., A. J. Bradshaw, et al. "Evaluation of a "nondieting" stress reduction program for overweight women: a randomized trial." *American Journal of Health Promotion* 22 (2008): 264–74.

Matthews, K. A., B. B. Gump, et al. "Hostile behaviors predict cardiovascular mortality among men enrolled in the Multiple Risk Factor Intervention Trial." *Circulation* 109 (2004): 66–70.

Naska, A., E. Oikonomou, A. Trichopoulou, T. Psaltopoulou, D. Trichopoulos. "Siesta in healthy adults and coronary mortality in the general population." *Archives of Internal Medicine* 167 (2007): 296–301.

Penson, R. T., R. A. Partridge, "Laughter: the best medicine?" *Oncologist* 10 (2005): 651–60.

Rainforth, M. V., R. H. Schneider, et al. "Stress Reduction Programs in Patients with Elevated Blood Pressure: A Systematic Review and Meta-analysis." *Current Hypertension Reports* 9 (2007): 520–8.

Schneider, R. H., C. N. Alexander, et al. "Long-term effects of stress reduction on mortality in persons > or = 55 years of age with systemic hypertension." *American Journal of Cardiology* 95 (2005): 1060–4.

Sivasankaran, S, S. Pollard-Quintner, et al. "The effect of a six-week program of yoga and meditation on brachial artery reactivity: do psychosocial interventions affect vascular tone?" *Clinical Cardiology* 29 (2006): 393–8.

Step 4: Take Command of Your Blood Pressure

Chobanian Aram V., George L. Bakris, Henry R. Black, William C. Cushman, Lee A. Green, Joseph L. Izzo, Jr, Daniel W. Jones, Barry J. Materson, Suzanne Oparil, Jackson T. Wright, Jr, Edward J. Roccella, and the National High Blood Pressure Education Program Coordinating Committee. "The Seventh Report of the Joint National Committee on Prevention, Detection, Evaluation, and Treatment of High Blood Pressure." *Journal of the American Medical Association* (2003): 289.

Fauci, Anthony S. *Harrison's Principles of Internal Medicine V1.* New York: McGraw-Hill Companies, The, 2008.

Izzo, Joseph L., ed. *Hypertension Primer: The Essentials of High Blood Pressure: Basic Science, Population Science, and Clinical Management.* Philadelphia: Lippincott Williams & Wilkins, 2007.

Libby, Peter, Robert O. Bonow, Douglas L. Mann, and Douglas P.

Zipes, eds. *Braunwald's Heart Disease: A Textbook of Cardiovascular Medicine*. Philadelphia: Saunders, 2007.

Murphy, Joseph G., ed. *Mayo Clinic Cardiology Review*. New York: Informa Healthcare, 2006.

Walsh, Richard A., Philip Poole-Wilson, and Spencer B. King, eds. *Hurst's the Heart*. New York: McGraw-Hill Professional, 2007.

Step 5: Control Your Cholesterol

"Detection, Evaluation, and Treatment of High Blood Cholesterol in Adults (Adult Treatment Panel III)." *National Heart Lung and Blood Institute*. 2004. <http://www.nhlbi.nih.gov/guidelines/cholesterol/>.

Fauci, Anthony S. *Harrison's Principles of Internal Medicine V1*. New York: McGraw-Hill Companies, The, 2008.

Murphy, Joseph G., ed. *Mayo Clinic Cardiology Review*. New York: Informa Healthcare, 2006.

Walsh, Richard A., Philip Poole-Wilson, and Spencer B. King, eds. *Hurst's the Heart*. New York: McGraw-Hill Professional, 2007.

Step 6: Reduce Free Radicals and Oxidative Stress

Adhami, V. M., A. Malik, et al. "Combined Inhibitory Effects of Green Tea Polyphenols and Selective Cyclooxygenase-2 Inhibitors on the Growth of Human Prostate Cancer Cells Both *In vitro* and *In vivo*." Clinical Cancer Research 13 (2007): 1611–1619.

Agusti, A., J. B. Soriano. "COPD as a Systemic Disease." *Chronic Obstructive Pulmonary Disease* 5 (2008): 133–8.

Ahmed, S., A. Pakozdi, et al. "Regulation of interleukin-1beta-induced chemokine production and matrix metalloproteinase 2 activation by epigallocatechin-3-gallate in rheumatoid arthritis synovial fibroblasts." *Arthritis & Rheumatism* 54 (2006): 2393–401.

Alyan, O., F. Kacmaz, et al. "Effects of Cigarette Smoking on Heart Rate Variability and Plasma N-Terminal Pro-B-Type Natriuretic Peptide in Healthy Subjects: Is There the Relationship between Both Markers?" *Annals of Noninvasive Electrocardiology* 13 (2008): 137–44.

Azadzoi, K. M., R. N. Schulman, et al. "Oxidative stress in arteriogenic erectile dysfunction: prophylactic role of antioxidants." *Journal of Urology* 174 (2005): 386–93.

Biswas, S., I. Rahman. "Modulation of steroid activity in chronic inflammation: A novel anti-inflammatory role for curcumin." *Molecular Nutrition & Food Research* (2008).

Bonomini, F., S. Tengattini, et al. "Atherosclerosis and oxidative stress." *Histology and Histopathology* 23 (2008): 381–90.

Brown, M. K., J. L. Evans, et al. "Beneficial effects of natural antioxidants EGCG and alpha-lipoic acid on life span and age-dependent behavioral declines in Caenorhabditis elegans." *Pharmacology, Biochemistry, and Behavior* 85 (2006): 620–8.

Engler, M. B., M. M. Engler, et al. "Flavonoid-rich dark chocolate improves endothelial function and increases plasma epicatechin concentrations in healthy adults." *Journal of the American College of Nutrition* 23 (2004): 197–204.

Forest, C. P., H. Padma-Nathan, H. R. Liker. "Efficacy and safety of pomegranate juice on improvement of erectile dysfunction in male patients with mild to moderate erectile dysfunction: a randomized, placebo-controlled, double-blind, crossover study." *International Journal of Impotence Research* 19 (2007): 564–7.

Gebhardt, Bear Jack. *The Enlightened Smoker's Guide to Quitting.* Dallas: BenBella Books, 2008.

Gerry, J. M., G. Pascual. "Narrowing in on Cardiovascular Disease: The Atheroprotective Role of Peroxisome Proliferator-Activated Receptor gamma." *Trends in Cardiovascular Medicine* 18 (2008): 39–44.

Goel, A., A. B. Kunnumakkara, B. B. Aggarwal. "Curcumin as "Curecumin": From kitchen to clinic." *Biochemical Pharmacology* 75 (2008): 787–809.

Gorelik, S., M. Ligumsky, et al. "A novel function of red wine polyphenols in humans: prevention of absorption of cytotoxic lipid peroxidation products." *Federation of American Societies for Experimental Biology Journal* 22 (2008): 41–6.

Harman, D. "Free radical theory of aging." *Mutation Research* 275 (1992): 257–66.

Hatcher, H., R. Planalp, et al. "Curcumin: From ancient medicine to current clinical trials." *Cellular and Molecular Life Sciences* (2008).

Higuera-Ciapara, I., L. Felix-Valenzuela, et al. "Astaxanthin: a review of its chemistry and applications." *Critical Reviews in Food Science and Nutrition* 46 (2006): 185–96.

Hussein, G., U. Sankawa, et al. "Astaxanthin, a carotenoid with potential in human health and nutrition." *Journal of Natural Products* 69 (2006): 443–9.

Ide, R., Y. Fujino, et al. "A Prospective Study of Green Tea Consumption and Oral Cancer Incidence in Japan." *Annals of Epidemiology* (2007).

Kuhn, H., P. Chaitidis, et al. "Arachidonic Acid metabolites in the cardiovascular system: the role of lipoxygenase isoforms in atherogenesis with particular emphasis on vascular remodeling." *Journal of Cardiovascular Pharmacology* 50 (2007): 609–20.

Lancaster, T., L. Stead. "Physician advice for smoking cessation." *Cochrane Database of Systematic Reviews* (2004).

Libby, P., P. M. Ridker, A. Maseri. "Inflammation and atherosclerosis." *Circulation* 105 (2002): 1135–43.

Lucini, D., F. Bertocchi, et al. "A controlled study of the autonomic changes produced by habitual cigarette smoking in healthy subjects." *Cardiovascular Research* 31 (1996): 633–9.

Murphy, M. P., R. A. Smith. "Targeting antioxidants to mitochondria by conjugation to lipophilic cations." *Annual Review of Pharmacology and Toxicology* 47 (2007): 629–56.

O'Keefe, J. H., N. M. Gheewala, J. O. O'Keefe. "Dietary strategies for improving post-prandial glucose, lipids, inflammation, and cardiovascular health." *Journal of the American College of Cardiology* 51 (2008): 249–55.

Papatheodorou, L., N. Weiss. "Vascular oxidant stress and inflammation in hyperhomocysteinemia." *Antioxidants and Redox Signaling* 9 (2007): 1941–58.

Prior, R. L., L. Gu, et al. "Plasma antioxidant capacity changes following a meal as a measure of the ability of a food to alter in vivo antioxidant status." *Journal of the American College of Nutrition* 26 (2007): 170–81.

Rizzo, M., E. Corrado, et al. "Prediction of cardio- and cerebrovascular events in patients with subclinical carotid atherosclerosis and low HDL-cholesterol." *Atherosclerosis* (2008).

Schleicher, E., U. Friess. "Oxidative stress, AGE, and atherosclerosis." *Kidney International Supplement* (2007): S17–26.

Seeram, N. P., M. Aviram, et al. "Comparison of Antioxidant Potency of Commonly Consumed Polyphenol-Rich Beverages in the United States." *Journal of Agriculture and Food Chemistry* 56 (2008): 1415–1422.

Son, S. M. "Role of vascular reactive oxygen species in development of vascular abnormalities in diabetes." *Diabetes Research and Clinical Practice* 77 (2007): S65–70.

Tan, K. T., G. Y. Lip. "Imaging of the unstable plaque." *International Journal of Cardiology* (2008).

Taubert, D., R. Roesen, et al. "Effects of low habitual cocoa intake on blood pressure and bioactive nitric oxide: a randomized controlled trial." *Journal of the American Medical Association* 298 (2007): 49–60.

Thangapazham, R. L., A. K. Singh, et al. "Green tea polyphenols and its constituent epigallocatechin gallate inhibits proliferation of human breast cancer cells in vitro and in vivo." *Cancer Letters* 245 (2007): 232–41.

Weinreb, O., S. Mandel, et al. "Neurological mechanisms of green tea polyphenols in Alzheimer's and Parkinson's diseases." *Journal of Nutritional Biochemistry* 15 (2004): 506–16.

Wolfram, S., D. Raederstorff, et al. "Epigallocatechin gallate supplementation alleviates diabetes in rodents." *Journal of Nutrition* 136 (2006): 2512–8.

Yamagishi, S., T. Matsui, K. Nakamura. "Possible involvement of tobacco-derived advanced glycation end products (AGEs) in an increased risk for developing cancers and cardiovascular disease in former smokers." *Medical Hypotheses* (2008).

Yasuda, O., Y. Takemura. "Aspirin: recent developments." *Cellular and Molecular Life Sciences* 65 (2008): 354–8.

Yusuf, N., C. Irby, et al. "Photoprotective effects of green tea polyphenols." *Photodermatology, Photoimmunology & Photomedicine* 23 (2007): 48–56.

Step 7: Avoid Chronic Inflammation

Charrier-Hisamuddin, L., C. L. Laboisse, D. Merlin. "ADAM-15: a metalloprotease that mediates inflammation." *Federation of American Societies for Experimental Biology Journal* 22 (2008): 641–53.

Chilton, F. H., L. L. Rudel. "Mechanisms by which botanical lipids affect inflammatory disorders." *American Journal of Clinical Nutrition* 87 (2008): 498S–503S.

Cipollone, F.,A. Mezzetti, et al. "Association between 5-lipoxygenase expression and plaque instability in humans." *Arteriosclerosis, Thrombosis, and Vascular Biology* 25 (2005): 1665–70.

Cuaz-Pérolin, C., Billiet, L., et al. "Antiinflammatory and antiatherogenic effects of the NF-kappaB inhibitor acetyl-11-keto-beta-boswellic acid in LPS-challenged ApoE-/- mice." *Arteriosclerosis, Thrombosis, and Vascular Biology* 28 (2008): 272–7.

Davis, D. R., J. H. Erlich. "Cardiac tissue factor: roles in physiology and fibrosis." *Clinical and Experimental Pharmacology and Physiology* 35 (2008): 342–8.

Erridge C. "The roles of pathogen-associated molecular patterns in atherosclerosis." *Trends in Cardiovascular Medicine* 18 (2008): 52–6.

Gawaz, M. "Platelets in the onset of atherosclerosis." *Blood Cells, Molecules, and Diseases* 36 (2006): 206–10.

Gerry, J. M., G. Pascual. "Narrowing in on Cardiovascular Disease: The Atheroprotective Role of Peroxisome Proliferator-Activated Receptor gamma." *Trends in Cardiovascular Medicine* 18 (2008): 39–44.

Libby, P. "Inflammatory mechanisms: the molecular basis of inflammation and disease." *Nutrition Review* 65 (2007) S140–6.

Libby, P, P. M. Ridker, A. Maseri. "Inflammation and atherosclerosis." *Circulation* 105 (2002): 1135–43.

May, A. E., P. Seizer, M. Gawaz. "Platelets: inflammatory firebugs of vascular walls." *Arteriosclerosis, Thrombosis, and Vascular Biology* 28 (2008): s5–10.

O'Keefe, J. H., N. M. Gheewala, J. O. O'Keefe. "Dietary strategies for improving post-prandial glucose, lipids, inflammation, and cardiovascular health." *Journal of the American College of Cardiology* 51 (2008): 249–55.

Packard, R. R., P. Libby. "Inflammation in atherosclerosis: from vascular biology to biomarker discovery and risk prediction." *Clinical Chemistry* 54 (2008): 24–38.

Singh, S., A. Khajuria, et al. "Boswellic acids: A leukotriene inhibitor also effective through topical application in inflammatory disorders." *Phytomedicine* (2008).

Smith, R. N., N. J. Mann, et al. "The effect of a high-protein, low glycemic-load diet versus a conventional, high glycemic-load diet on biochemical parameters associated with acne vulgaris: a randomized, investigator-masked, controlled trial." *Journal of the American Academy of Dermatology* 57 (2007): 247–56.

Yasuda, O., Y. Takemura, et al. "Aspirin: recent developments." *Cellular and Molecular Life Sciences* 65 (2008): 354–8.

Step 8: Prevent Metabolic Syndrome and Diabetes

Alexander, C. M., P. B. Landsman, S. M. Grundy. "The influence of age and body mass index on the metabolic syndrome and its components." *Diabetes, Obesity, and Metabolism* 10 (2008): 246–50.

Alizadeh Dehnavi, R., E. D. Beishuizen, et al. "The impact of metabolic syndrome and CRP on vascular phenotype in type 2 diabetes mellitus." *European Journal of Internal Medicine* 19 (2008): 115–21.

Aronson, D. "Hyperglycemia and the pathobiology of diabetic complications." *Advanced Cardiology* 45 (2008): 1–16.

Barnard, R. J. "Prostate cancer prevention by nutritional means to alleviate metabolic syndrome." *American Journal of Clinical Nutrition* 86 (2007): S889–93.

Cao, J. J., A. M. Arnold, et al. "Association of carotid artery intima-media thickness, plaques, and C-reactive protein with future cardiovascular disease and all-cause mortality: the Cardiovascular Health Study." *Circulation* 116 (2007): 32–8.

Hamburg, N. M., C. J. McMackin, et al. "Physical inactivity rapidly induces insulin resistance and microvascular dysfunction in healthy volunteers." *Arteriosclerosis, Thrombosis, and Vascular Biology* 27 (2007): 2650–6.

Hsu, I. R., S. P. Kim, et al. "Metabolic syndrome, hyperinsulinemia, and cancer." *American Journal of Clinical Nutrition* 86 (2007): S867–71.

Imig, J. D. "Eicosanoids and renal damage in cardiometabolic syndrome." *Expert Opinion on Drug Metabolism and Toxicology* 4 (2008): 165–74.

O'Keefe, J. H., N. M. Gheewala, J. O. O'Keefe. "Dietary strategies for improving post-prandial glucose, lipids, inflammation, and cardiovascular health." *Journal of the American College of Cardiology* 51 (2008): 249–55.

Rammos, G., P. Tseke, S. Ziakka. "Vitamin D, the renin-angiotensin system, and insulin resistance." *International Urology and Nephrology* (2008).

Reaven, Gerald M., Terry Kristen Strom, and Barry Fox. *Syndrome X, the Silent Killer: The New Heart Disease Risk*. New York: Simon & Schuster, 2001.

Schiffrin, E. L., M. L. Lipman, J. F. Mann. "Chronic kidney disease: effects on the cardiovascular system." *Circulation* 116 (2007): 85–97.

Son, S. M. "Role of vascular reactive oxygen species in development of vascular abnormalities in diabetes." *Diabetes Research and Clinical Practice* (2007): S65–70.

You, T., B. J. Nicklas, et al. "The Metabolic Syndrome Is Associated With Circulating Adipokines in Older Adults Across a Wide Range of Adiposity." *Journals of Gerontology Series A: Biological Sciences and Medical Sciences* 63 (2008): 414–419.

Step 9: Have an Annual Physical Exam with Comprehensive Lab

Kulkarni, K. R. "Cholesterol profile measurement by vertical auto profile method." *Clinical Laboratory Language* 26 (2006): 787–802.

Mudd, J. O., B. A. Borlaug, et al. "Beyond low-density lipoprotein cholesterol: defining the role of low-density lipoprotein heterogeneity in coronary artery disease." *Journal of the American College of Cardiology* 50 (2007): 1735–41.

Ozner, M. "VAP Cholesterol Testing. Advanced technology uncovers hidden cardiovascular risks." *Life Extension Magazine*, May 2007.

Superko, H. R. "Did grandma give you heart disease? The new battle against coronary artery disease." *American Journal of Cardiology* 82 (1998): 34–46.

Ziajka, P. "Using VAP expanded lipid testing from Atherotec to develop optimal patient treatment plans (Third Edition)." *American Journal of Cardiology* 82 (1998): 34Q.

Step 10: Avoid Unnecessary Diagnostic Tests and Procedures

"Body Scans. Do you know the risk?": *Life Extension*, November 2001.

Brenner, D. J., C. D. Elliston. "Estimated radiation risks potentially associated with full-body CT screening." *Radiology* 232 (2004): 735–8.

Brenner, D. J., E. J. Hall. "Computed tomography—an increasing source of radiation exposure." New England Journal of Medicine 357 (2007): 2277–84.

Brody, J. E. "Personal health; how perils can await the worried wealthy." *New York Times*, 12 Nov. 2002.

Clark, C. "Latest scanning device finds heart disease, and controversy, quickly." *San Diego Union-Tribune*, 1 Oct. 2006.

Coles, D. R., M. A. Smail, I. S. Negus, et al. "Comparison of radiation doses from multislice computed tomography coronary angiography and conventional diagnostic angiography." *Journal of the American College of Cardiology* 47 (2006): 1840–5.

Einstein, A. J., M. J. Henzlova, S. Rajagopalan. "Estimating risk of cancer associated with radiation exposure from 64-slice computed tomography coronary angiography." *Journal of the American Medical Association* 298 (2007): 317–23.

Gorman, C. "How new heart-scanning technology could save your life." *Time*, 28 August 2005.

Hall, E. J., D. J. Brenner. "Cancer risks from diagnostic radiology." *British Journal of Radiology* 81 (2008): 362–78.

Kalayoglu, Murat V. "64-slice CT and the New Age for Cardiac Diagnostics." *Medcompare*. 7 Nov. 2007.

Kolata, G. "Heart scanner stirs new hope and a debate." *New York Times*, 17 Nov. 2004.

Masters, C. "Should you have a CT scan?" *Time*. 17 July 2007.

Mollet, N. R., F. Cademartiri, C. A. van Mieghem, et al. "High-resolution spiral computed tomography coronary angiography in patients referred for diagnostic conventional coronary angiography." *Circulation* 112 (2005): 2318–23.

Nainggolan, L. "Stress echo identifies women at highest risk for CAD." *Heartwire*, 17 June 2007.

O'Malley, P. G., I. M. Feuerstein, A. J. Taylor. "Impact of electron beam tomography, with or without case management, on motivation, behavioral change, and cardiovascular risk profile: a randomized controlled trial." *Journal of the American Medical Association* 289 (2003): 2215–23.

Ozner, M. "Avoiding the Radiation Dangers of Cardiac CAT Scans." *Life Extension Magazine*, March 2008.

Rabin, R. C. "The consumer: with rise in radiation exposure, experts urge caution on tests." *New York Times*, 19 June 2007.

Redberg, R. F. "Computed tomographic angiography: more than just a pretty picture?" *Journal of the American College of Cardiology* 49 (2007): 1827–9.

Waugh, N., C. Black, et al. "The effectiveness and cost-effectiveness of computed tomography screening for coronary artery disease: systematic review." *Health Technology Assessment* 10 (2006): iii-iv, ix–x, 1–41.

Index

About the Author

MICHAEL OZNER, MD, FACC, FAHA, is one of America's leading advocates for heart disease prevention. Dr. Ozner is a board-certified cardiologist, a Fellow of the American College of Cardiology and of the American Heart Association, medical director of Wellness & Prevention at Baptist Health South Florida, and a well-known regional and national speaker in the field of preventive cardiology. He is the medical director of the Cardiovascular Prevention Institute of South Florida and symposium director for "Cardiovascular Disease Prevention," an annual international meeting highlighting advances in preventive cardiology. He was the recipient of the 2008 American Heart Association Humanitarian Award. Dr. Ozner is also the author of the BenBella Books title *The Miami Mediterranean Diet*.

To contact Dr. Michael Ozner: www.drozner.com